T0264957

"Ingrid Pénzes is an experienced art therapist who completed her doctoral research on the role of art materials in art therapy assessment in the Netherlands. This book is a clear and succinct summary of how her way of assessing has been influenced by this research and provides a rich resource for fellow art therapy practitioners and trainees to use in their practice. For once, dissemination of research findings has been clearly adapted and presented for practice."

Ditty Dokter, *PhD. Codarts Rotterdam, The Netherlands and Anglia Ruskin University, Cambridge, UK*

"This is what art therapy needs. The art form as the foundation of our profession, scientifically proven and cast in a clear assessment tool. ArTA is without a doubt a new standard for practice and education."

Sanne Van Gelder, *MA, Art Therapist and Training Coordinator BaNaBa Creative Therapy PXL University of Applied Sciences Hasselt, Belgium*

"An exciting book in many ways. Once we thought we could understand people by having them look at drawings, then came the time when we looked at their drawings, and now Ingrid Pénzes prepares us for the next step: it's not about what someone draws, but how someone draws. The ArTA method systematically searches for the signs of health: 'What do you need to come into your power?'"

Giel Hutschemaekers, *Professor of Mental Health Care, Radboud University Nijmegen, The Netherlands*

Art Therapy Observation and Assessment in Clinical Practice

This book describes ArTA, an evidence-based method for art therapy observation and assessment. This novel method argues the art-making process and art product are related to aspects of mental health. The results of the author's own research show that observed patterns in material interaction, material experience, and the specific combinations of formal elements of the art product reveal the client's balance between thinking and feeling, and adaptability. Divided into four sections, the book illustrates this research, theory, and application of the ArTA method using examples and case histories with clear frameworks that give guidance in art therapy observation and assessment. It provides direction for formulating treatment goals and drawing up appropriate treatment interventions. Intended for art therapy students and practicing art therapists, this methodology will challenge readers to rethink the relationship between a client's interaction with art materials and their mental health.

Ingrid Pénzes is an art therapist, mental health scientist, and Doctor of Social Sciences. She holds a doctorate in the relationship between the art form and mental health. She has worked at the intersection of art therapy education, practice, and science for many years. To translate scientific knowledge into education and practice, she offers training, research, and assessment for institutions, companies, and professionals.

Art Therapy Observation and Assessment in Clinical Practice

The ArTA Method

Ingrid Pénzes

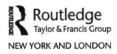

Routledge
Taylor & Francis Group

NEW YORK AND LONDON

Designed cover image: by Ingrid Pénzes

First published 2024
by Routledge
605 Third Avenue, New York, NY 10158

and by Routledge
4 Park Square, Milton Park, Abingdon, Oxon, OX14 4RN

Routledge is an imprint of the Taylor & Francis Group, an informa business

© 2024 Ingrid Pénzes

The right of Ingrid Pénzes to be identified as author of this work has been asserted in accordance with sections 77 and 78 of the Copyright, Designs and Patents Act 1988.

All rights reserved. No part of this book may be reprinted or reproduced or utilised in any form or by any electronic, mechanical, or other means, now known or hereafter invented, including photocopying and recording, or in any information storage or retrieval system, without permission in writing from the publishers.

Trademark notice: Product or corporate names may be trademarks or registered trademarks, and are used only for identification and explanation without intent to infringe.

ISBN: 9781032549637 (hbk)
ISBN: 9781032549613 (pbk)
ISBN: 9781003428305 (ebk)

DOI: 10.4324/9781003428305

Typeset in Times New Roman
by codeMantra

For Anja

Contents

Foreword   *xi*
LISA D. HINZ

Preface   *xiii*

1   ArTA: the basics   1
Introduction 1
1.1   Art therapy 1
1.2   The art therapy triangle 2
1.3   The context of art-making: coherence of material,
        technique, and instruction 4
        1.3.1   Art material 6
        1.3.2   Technique and tools 6
        1.3.3   Instruction 8
1.4   Mental health 10
        1.4.1   Balance 12
        1.4.2   Adaptability 13
1.5   Neuroanalogous processes 14
        1.5.1   A neuroscientific approach to health 15
        1.5.2   Analogies between neurological processes
                 and art-making 17

2   ArTA: the theory   29
Introduction 29
2.1   The evidence base of ArTA 30
2.2   A little history 34
2.3   ArTA 39
2.4   Material interaction 39
        2.4.1   Style of material interaction 41
        2.4.2   Patterns of material Interaction 42

2.5   *Material experience 44*
2.6   *Art product 45*
    2.6.1   Formal elements 46
    2.6.2   Structure 51
    2.6.3   Variation 53
2.7   *Relationship between material interaction, material experience, and art product 56*
2.8   *The relationship between material interaction, material experience, art product, and mental health 59*
2.9   *Role of instruction 61*
2.10   *Role of reflection 66*
2.11   *Role of the therapeutic relationship 68*
2.12   *Indication 69*

3   ArTA: the methodical application   **77**
Introduction 77
3.1   *The ArTA observation form 77*
3.2   *The four steps of ArTA 79*
    3.2.1   Step 1: Observing 79
    3.2.2   Step 2: Analyzing 82
    3.2.3   Step 3: Interpreting 84
    3.2.4   Step 4: Formulating 86

4   ArTA: a case description   **88**
Introduction 88
4.1   *Case 89*
4.2   *Observations during observation session 1 89*
4.3   *Observations during observation session 2 90*
4.4   *Observations during session 3: accompanying observation session 1 91*
4.5   *Observations during session 4: observation session 3 92*
4.6   *Findings during the overall reflection 94*

Epilogue   *108*
Appendix 1: extended definitions of formal elements of art products on a five-point scale   *111*
Appendix 2: ArTA observation form   *117*
Index   *125*

Foreword

Since its beginnings, the field of art therapy has struggled to find a form of visual analysis that supports art therapy assessment as well as articulates a connection between the assessment of art produced in session and the formulation of treatment goals. Various methods have been borrowed from psychology or created within the field, but all have been criticized and none has been universally adopted.

With the creation of the Art Therapy Assessment (ArTA), Dr. Ingrid Pénzes has constructed a sophisticated and comprehensive evaluative system that draws from her vast research experience on material interaction, material experience, and the relationship between art product and process and mental health. ArTA is rooted in the history of art therapy and the various ways that art assessment has been approached over time. In addition, it includes up-to-date information about the influence of the art therapy triad and other factors on the assessment process.

ArTA is a method of analysis firmly grounded in art therapy: the importance of art materials, artistic methods, and the relationship between the art therapist and client all are considered. Pénzes highlights the ways in which the processes that influence material interaction in art therapy are analogous to the processes that impact behavior in other areas of life. This is the basis for art assessment and its relationship to the establishment of treatment goals. ArTA can help art therapists develop a language to articulate what occurs in the art therapy session – even beyond the assessment phase – and how these events are related to other aspects of the client's life, especially in relation to balance and adaptability.

Pénzes' ArTA approach to formulating treatment goals is based upon a joint reflection on the assessment process and art products by the client and art therapist. In this way, the assessment takes into account that each person interacts with materials in a unique way given the structure of their nervous system. It aids in the formulation of treatment goals that are realistic and tailored to the individual client.

The process of the art therapy assessment is first grounded in history and theory and then explained in a step-by-step fashion. ArTA is further brought to life through an in-depth analysis of a clinical case, from an explanation of the initial material interaction to the client's material experience, and an exploration of the art products. The relationship between the assessment of these three variables and the establishment of treatment goals is clearly laid out and supported by clear examples, charts, and illustrations.

It is obvious on first reading, that ArTA is based on many years of research, data analysis and clinical work. This comprehensive study of material interaction and its place in art assessment will greatly help students and new art therapists gain insight into how assessment and treatment occur and are related to one another in art therapy. Further, it will provide structure and validation to the experiences and observations of seasoned art therapists.

I know that this is a book that the reader will refer to countless times over the years.

Lisa D. Hinz, Ph.D., ATR-BC
Associate Professor of Art Therapy Psychology
Dominican University of California
San Rafael, California, USA

Preface

This book describes the ArTA (Art Therapy Assessment) method. ArTA is an evidence-based assessment, developed based on the findings of my doctoral research. As an art therapist and having worked as an art therapy teacher for many years, my main motivation was to translate the scientific insights of my research into practice and education.

As an art therapist and a psychologist, I am convinced that a thorough art therapy assessment is the foundation for further treatment. It helps gain insight into the client's needs – both challenges and strengths. It aids in determining whether art therapy is an appropriate form of treatment for the client, and if so, what treatment goals can be formulated and what art therapy interventions can be used to work toward those goals.

The results of the ArTA research show that it is not so much *what* someone makes in art therapy, but more importantly, *how* someone makes it. How the client interacts with the art material – the so-called material interaction – becomes tangible – the so-called "material experience" – and visible in the art product. The specific combination of reliably observable formal elements – movement, dynamics, contour, repetition, mixture of color, and color saturation – determines the structure and variation of an art product. And that structure and variation say something about the mental health of the creator. Not so much in terms of illness and what is wrong, but primarily in terms of the balance between thinking and feeling, and the power and ability to improve, or adaptability.

ArTA adopts a neuro-analogical model of thinking and, therefore, assumes that the processes that drive everyday functioning are the same processes that are activated in the art-making process in art therapy. ArTA can be used to identify how someone copes with challenging situations, and the potential for increasing adaptability. ArTA can be used at the beginning of art therapy as well as during treatment to monitor progress. This assessment is widely applicable to assess adults with a variety of mental health problems.

ArTA is widely applicable because a large number of art therapists from different countries, working with various art therapy methodologies, and an even larger number of clients with diverse needs in adult mental health care participated in the study. ArTA, therefore, transcends different art therapy approaches and mental health problems.

To properly understand and apply the ArTA method, it is important to first become familiar with the ArTA conceptual framework. This is the foundation of the method, and this is where the book begins. In Chapter 1, these concepts are described and explained. The art therapy triangle is discussed, and mental health is addressed. The relationship between mental health and the art form is also featured. I will also describe the therapeutic effects of the experiential use of art materials, techniques, and the instructions for art-making.

In Chapter 2, the theory that underlies the ArTA method is described. This chapter begins with a summary of the research underlying ArTA followed by a brief historical overview of art therapy observation and assessment. This shows that the international landscape of art therapy assessment is enormously diverse. How does ArTA fit in? The three main pillars of ArTA observation are then discussed: "material interaction," "material experience," and "art product." I also explain how these pillars are interrelated and can be interpreted in terms of "balance" and "adaptability" as aspects of mental health.

The methodical application of ArTA, in particular the four steps of observing, analyzing, interpreting, and formulating, is described in Chapter 3. It is important to emphasize that ArTA is not a "cookbook," as the method cannot be applied without professional art therapy training and expertise. The steps provide guidance for making evidence-based diagnostic statements about adult clients. These art therapy findings help determine whether a client could benefit from art therapy. And, if so, what the focus of treatment might be, what treatment goals can be formulated, and what art therapy interventions can be employed that contribute to the client's health.

In Chapter 4, the method with a case study is illustrated. We meet Yasper and go through the four steps of ArTA. On this basis, the ArTA Observation Form is completed, making the application of ArTA concrete.

The ArTA observation form is also attached as Appendix 2. Please note that the observation form is only a tool for practicing the ArTA method. It cannot be viewed and used in isolation from the underlying theory and expertise of the art therapist. Once you have mastered the method, you certainly do not need to fill out this form for every client. It would take too much time.

Because training, in addition to this book, helps to master the method, the form is used in the ArTA Basic Course. After training, you will find that you no longer need to analyze and note all the components on the form. A trained eye can quickly see, for example, whether the material interaction is rational or affective, and the degree of structure and variation in an art product. Once the method is mastered to this degree, an abbreviated version of the form can be used. This saves a lot of work and time in an already busy clinical practice!

Chapter 1

ArTA
The basics

Introduction

To properly understand and apply the ArTA method, it is important to first become familiar with the ArTA basics. This is the foundation of the method, and this is where the book begins. This chapter describes how art therapy and mental health, including the concepts of balance and adaptability, are considered in ArTA. It discusses what is meant by art therapy, mental health, the art therapy triangle, the art form (including the role of art materials, techniques and tools, and instruction), and the importance of experiential work from a neuroanalogical thinking model.[1] This includes a neuroscientific perspective on health and the analogy between the processes that drive daily functioning and art making in art therapy. It theorizes how the methodical use of the combination of art materials, techniques, tools, and instructions – the so-called art therapy mixing panel – affects the structure and thus the experience of the art-making process. At the end of this chapter, you will have sufficient knowledge of these basic concepts within ArTA.

1.1 Art therapy

Internationally, art therapists work from a variety of approaches (see §2.2). As a result, different descriptions and definitions of art therapy can be found in the literature.[2] Within ArTA, art therapy is defined as follows:

Art therapy is an action- and experience-oriented form of therapy in which a professionally trained art therapist methodically uses interventions with art materials, tools, techniques, and instructions to initiate change tailored to the client that contributes to mental health.

The methodical use of art materials in an art-making process results in an art product. This distinguishes art therapy from other more verbal forms of therapy. The art form is used methodically to provide clients with physical, sensory, emotional, and cognitive experiences that enable them to shape a process of change, development, stabilization, or acceptance. These processes affect emotional, behavioral, cognitive, social, neurological, and/or physical aspects of functioning.

DOI: 10.4324/9781003428305-1

The (neuropsychological) processes activated during art-making are analogous to the processes that drive our (daily) functioning. Through the methodical use of the art form, clients gain experiences that have an impact on these processes and thus contribute to their mental health.

Within ArTA, the methodical use of the art form is considered essential. The art form is what distinguishes art therapy from other arts therapies and other forms of treatment. Together with the client and the therapist, the art form completes the art therapy triangle.

1.2   The art therapy triangle

The art therapist uses the art form as a therapeutic tool: interacting with art material in an art-making process resulting in an art product. The art form is the third dimension of art therapy and, together with the client and the therapist, forms the art therapy triangle (see Figure 1.1).

Different art therapy approaches explain this triangle in their own way and emphasize different aspects (see §2.2). Within ArTA, the different angles and the relationship between them are considered as follows:

The *client* is an individual with a unique background, character, living conditions, and preferences. The client seeks help, often in response to complaints that interfere with functioning in daily life. Based on the severity of the complaints, the degree of impairment, and certainly the client's abilities, the therapist methodically uses the art form to shape the treatment. It is therefore important for the therapist to gain insight into these aspects of the client through observation and assessment.

The *therapist* is a specially trained professional who methodically uses the art form to initiate therapeutic processes aimed at achieving the client's individual

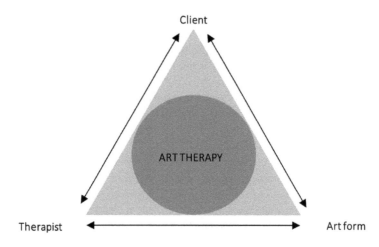

Figure 1.1 The art therapy triangle.

treatment goals. To do this, the therapist has theoretical knowledge of the psychotherapeutic effects of the art form, a broad repertoire of art-making skills, and mastery of various levels of creativity. The therapist also has therapeutic skills, such as listening and questioning, and therapeutic attitudes, such as showing compassion, being authentic, and offering support (see also §2.11).

The *art form* refers to the art materials and techniques methodically applied by the therapist and/or chosen by the client in an art-making process that results in an art product. This distinguishes art therapy and art therapy observation and assessment from other therapies.[3] Art materials have different characteristics. Some are solid in nature and therefore easier to control, such as most graphic materials. Others are fluid in nature and therefore less easily controlled, such as ink and watercolor. Art materials can be used with various techniques and associated tools to initiate change processes in therapy.[4] The art product is the visible and tangible result of the art-making process, such as a drawing, painting, or sculpture. An art product is permanent; it can be touched, observed, and analyzed. This provides an entry point for (shared) reflection and communication (see §2.10).

All corners of the triangle – the client, the therapist, and the art form – are important and they interact and influence each other. The arrows in Figure 1.3 represent these interactions. In art therapy practice, all corners interact simultaneously. This defines a session, a treatment phase, and the overall treatment. In attempting to reduce and understand this complexity, we unravel, somewhat artificially, the interaction between the different angles.

The arrow *therapist – art form* concerns the way in which the art therapist methodically employs the art form for the purposes of observation, assessment, and treatment. The properties of the material and technique ensure that the therapist makes appropriate choices based on his or her knowledge and expertise.

The *therapist – client* arrow refers to both verbal and nonverbal communication between the client and the therapist. Each brings their own frame of reference to the interaction so that the interaction is determined by this mutual influence. The therapist's task is to be present in a way that supports the client in the treatment process (see also §2.11).

The arrow *art form – client* refers to the interaction between the art form and the client. During the active working phase, the properties of the material and the technique influence the client. They invite them to react in a certain way,[5] such as wood invites to saw and a pencil to draw. And they evoke a personal experience (the so-called material experience, as pleasant, dirty, or frustrating, see §2.5). The client responds by interacting with the material in their own way (material interaction, see §2.4), resulting in an art product (see §2.6). This art product influences the client; it reminds them of their own experiences during the creative process and helps them to reflect on their choices. The client deals with it in their own way, for example by appreciating, valuing, or destroying it.

The art form thus adds an additional and distinctive dimension to art therapy. The methodical use of the art form is central within the art therapy treatment, and also within ArTA. Therefore, we will elaborate on this corner of the triangle.

1.3 The context of art-making: coherence of material, technique, and instruction

The art-making process in art therapy and in ArTA amounts to constructing an item; something is made. Depending on what is made, with what material, and how it is made, the art-making process has more or less structure. Structure refers to the degree of control and direction. Depending on the phase and goal of the treatment, the art therapist will provide more or less structure and thus determine the context of the session (see Figure 1.2). In order to determine the level of structure in an art therapy session, the art therapist uses a combination of

1   Art materials
2   Techniques and tools
3   Instruction

An example

An art therapist instructs a client to draw a portrait of someone. The technique used is memory-based drawing. The material used is a HB pencil on A4 paper (8-1/4 × 11-3/4 inches). The instructions are not complex or elaborate because they do not require a great number of steps to be memorized. Additionally, when

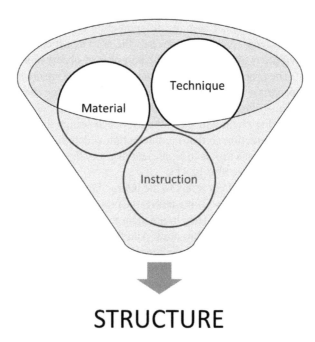

Figure 1.2 The combination of material, technique, and instruction determines the structure of the art therapy context.

it comes to drawing a portrait, most people have an idea of what is intended. Pencil drawing is usually familiar and offers a lot of guidance, making it easy for the client to control. In short, with this combination of material, technique, and instruction, the art therapist provides a relatively large amount of structure.[6]

Now suppose this art therapist adjusts the technique slightly: the portrait is not drawn from memory but redrawn from an example. This increases structure because the technique of copying from an example provides more guidance than drawing the portrait from memory.

On the other hand, the art therapist can also provide less structure based on instruction, materials, and technique.

An example

The art therapist instructs a client to create a free composition. The material used is watercolor on A3 paper (11.7 × 16.5 inches), and the technique is painting with a thick brush. The instruction is not complex or elaborate, but most people will not have an immediate idea when making a free composition. Moreover, watercolor is a material that flows easily, especially when combined with a thick brush, making it less easy to control. With this combination of material, technique, and instruction, the art therapist provides relatively little structure compared to the task of drawing a portrait with a pencil.

You may have noticed that the word "relatively" has been used several times. That is because there are many nuances in both the material, technique, and/ or tools and the instruction that determine the structure. For example, consider how much structure would be provided if the art therapist gave a client an assignment of free composition using watercolor and a thick brush, but on much larger paper? And if that paper was also made wet first? And without gluing this paper to a surface that would cause it to wobble? Or if the art therapist gave the client ten different materials, sizes, and types of paper to choose from, and the task was for the client to decide what to do.... The structure would be extremely reduced.

And how much structure would it provide if the art therapist instructed the client to paint a seascape in watercolor with a thick brush on A4 paper (8-1/4 × 11-3/4 inches), drawing lines from left to right in blue? On thick watercolor paper glued to a base? And the art therapist provided a quick demonstration... The structure would increase.

In short, the structure of the art-making process is determined by the combination of material, technique and tools, and instruction. Think of it as a kind of "mixing panel" with three buttons (material, technique and tools, and instruction) available to the art therapist to determine the structure of the art-making process in a session (see also Figure 1.8). This is a complex and nuanced interplay that requires skill and expertise on the part of the art therapist to match the structure to the individual client's treatment goals. It may be helpful to peel back some of this complexity and artificially separate the three components of material, technique and tools, and instruction

1.3.1 Art material

Art therapy involves working with the full range of two- and three-dimensional (2D and 3D) art materials: from pencil, crayon, ink, and paint to stone and clay. ArTA focusses mainly on working with 2D materials. The main reason for this is that the large number of art therapists who participated in the research on which ArTA is based worked primarily with two-dimensional materials in the context of observation and assessment. Material interaction and material experience are also involved when working with 3D materials although a category of material interaction such as "color mixing" may not apply. In a spatial art product, other formal elements may play a role in determining the structure and the variation. This simply requires further research. Therefore, in the context of ArTA, we focus on 2D materials.

Two-dimensional art materials have different properties, which we can roughly place on a continuum from solid to fluid. A pencil, for example, has completely different physical properties than colored ink. Solid materials give more grip than more fluid materials. Solid materials usually require some force, are usually dry, and are easier to control than fluid materials. Fluid materials are less easy to control but are easier to mix. The more solid a material is, the more structure it provides.

If we were to place art materials on a continuum from solid to fluid in terms of the degree of structure they provide solely on the basis of their physical properties and independent of their technique and tools, it would look like Figure 1.3.

However, the structure of the art-making process does not depend only on the properties of the art material; it is also influenced by technique and tools.

1.3.2 Technique and tools

It is not only the physical properties of the art material that affect structure. The technique used and the tools required also influence the degree of structure.

An example

Ink is a fluid material. When used with a fountain pen to draw or shade, for example, it offers more structure than when it is used with a bamboo brush and wet-on-wet technique. With the former technique, the creator has much more control, can work with more precision, can control the material, and has more grip than with the latter technique, where the fluidity of the ink is exacerbated by the technique, which offers little control and direction.

Or compare painting with acrylic paint with a small brush to painting with a coarse brush or spatula. The amount of water/medium added also plays a role in the structure created; water-based paints such as acrylic, gouache, and water-color become more fluid when mixed with a lot of water and remain more solid when mixed with less water.

Techniques involving different (supported) materials can also affect structure. For example, if colored ink is applied to a sheet of paper that has previously

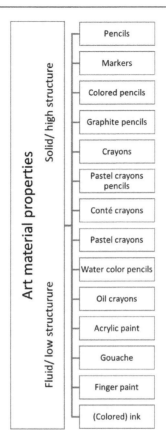

Figure 1.3 Properties of 2D materials arranged from solid to fluid and in relation to high and low structure.

been divided into sections with glue or tape, this will provide more support and
structure than if it is dripped onto a wet sheet.

From the above descriptions of techniques, it can be seen that 2D techniques
and tools can be placed on a continuum from linear (drawing/graphic), such as
drawing, sketching, shading, coloring, etc., to pictorial (painterly), such as painting, smearing, blending, flowing, dripping, etc. (see Figure 1.4).

Linear techniques tend to add more structure to the art-making process, while
pictorial techniques tend to add less structure.

The way the technique is used also matters; it makes a difference if you shade
slowly, and with precision, or if you do it at a fast pace from a free wrist. It also
makes a difference if the shading is done with one finger or the whole hand, or
even both. In the former cases, there will be more structure in the art-making
process than in the latter. The art therapist can encourage this by giving instructions. This is the third component that affects structure.

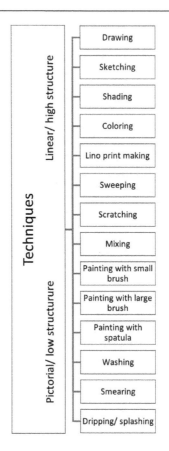

Figure 1.4 Techniques arranged from linear to pictorial and in relation to high and low structure.

1.3.3 Instruction

The instruction given also influences the structure of the art-making process. This depends on the complexity and degree of the instruction.[7]

The complexity of the instruction determines the number of actions to be performed. A high-complexity instruction usually contains many steps that need to be memorized, usually in a specific order, and leading to a specific result, such as drawing your parents' house at a scale of 1:100, or making a 6 × 6 inch linoleum print consisting of 10 layers. Low-complexity instructions usually involve fewer or no steps and do not require a specific outcome, such as making a random line drawing with any material you choose. An art therapist can vary the level of complexity by working with themes, for example.

The degree of instruction determines the freedom of choice given. With a low degree of instruction, the freedom of choice is great; with a high degree of

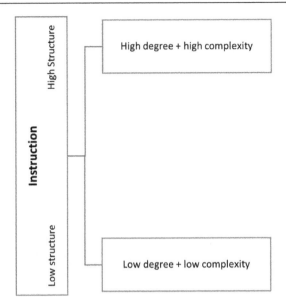

Figure 1.5 Instruction arranged from high to low level and in relation to high and low structure.

instruction, the freedom of choice is limited and a specific action and/or result is expected. An art therapist can vary the level of instruction by determining many or fewer factors such as whether or not to prescribe materials, technique, and format.

Based on the complexity and level, instruction can be placed on a continuum from high to low. High-level instruction consists of high complexity and degree of instruction: a specific result or action is expected, with a large number of steps that should be performed in a particular order. Low-level instruction consists of low complexity and degree of instruction: there is a wide range of choices with no specific end result or action expected.

The lower the level of instruction, the more freedom of choice, the more experimental the work process. In general, a high level of instruction tends to contribute to more structure in the art-making process, and a low level of instruction tends to contribute to less structure (see Figure 1.5).

In summary, structure in the art-making process is determined by the combination of material (solid-fluid), technique and tools (linear-pictorial), and level of instruction (high-low).

Art therapists have a sort of "mixing panel" at their disposal (see Figure 1.6).

Figure 1.6 shows the continua of materials, techniques and tools, and instruction, as discussed and illustrated above, in a horizontal direction. The open circles represent the buttons that can be moved fluidly across these continua. The specific combinations thus created define the structure in the art-making process.

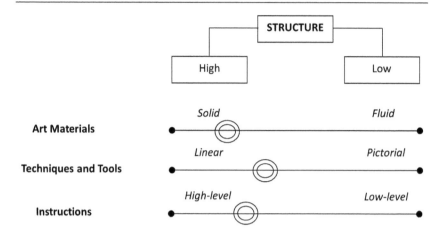

Figure 1.6 The art therapist's "mixing panel": the combination of properties of material, techniques and tools, and instruction determine the structure of art-making.

The combinations are almost limitless and require knowledge, skills, and expertise to apply methodically. The goal is always to improve the client's mental health.

1.4   Mental health

Just as there are different approaches to art therapy, there are different views of mental health. A full account of these is beyond the scope of this book, but broadly they can be divided into two approaches.

The first approach defines mental health in terms of "illness." Symptoms of disorders are classified in, for example, the Diagnostic and Statistical Manual of Mental Disorders (DSM, American Psychiatric Association [APA], 2013). Within this view, much attention is paid to factors related to the development and maintenance of psychopathology. This is also referred to as pathogenesis. It also includes the transdiagnostic approach (van Heycop ten Ham et al., 2014). Whereas the DSM classifies illnesses into disorders based on symptoms, the transdiagnostic approach assumes that different disorders have the same underlying mechanisms, such as disturbances in self-image and emotion regulation, perfectionism, and obsessive-compulsive behavior. Thus, different mechanisms may lead to or perpetuate different disorders.

An advantage of a classification system like the DSM is that it provides a common language for researchers. However, criticism of the DSM has increased in recent years. In particular, the criticism is that clients in clinical practice regularly deviate from the criteria used. Sometimes clients conform to more criteria that are outside the diagnosis than those within it. Often they display criteria that indicate multiple diagnoses. A system of care based on such classifications can therefore create situations in which the client receives unnecessary medication or, in the worst case, does not receive the most appropriate treatment.[8] In response to this medical-centered approach, the second approach is gaining ground.

The second approach defines mental health in terms of "health." This approach argues that mental health does not depend solely on the absence of symptoms and complaints, but that individuals always have healthy aspects even when they have symptoms. Therefore, according to this approach, it is not so much whether people have complaints or not, but how they deal with them. As early as 1979, Antonovsky emphasized the importance of factors that contribute to health rather than illness. He called this salutogenesis. He opposed the medical model and its dichotomy between sick and healthy. He was convinced that every human being, even when ill, has a healthy aspect. He saw the will to grow and develop as a force that should be addressed in treatment. This is in line with how the World Health Organization (WHO, 2021) defines health:

Health is a state of complete physical, mental and social well-being and not merely the absence of disease or infirmity. An important implication of this definition is that mental health is more than just the absence of mental disorders or disabilities. Mental health is a state of well-being in which an individual realizes his or her own abilities, can cope with the normal stresses of life, can work productively and is able to make a contribution to his or her community. Mental health is fundamental to our collective and individual ability as humans to think, emote, interact with each other, earn a living and enjoy life.

The focus on the healthy part fits seamlessly with Huber et al.'s (2016, p. 2) definition of positive health: *"[...] the ability to adapt and take personal control in the face of life's physical, emotional, and social challenges."* It emphasizes positive aspects of health such as psychological flexibility, mental resilience, and self-management. The main criticism of this approach is that this definition of health places too much emphasis on client autonomy, self-organization, and responsibility – even for clients who are (temporarily) unable to take on this responsibility due to the severity or complexity of their symptoms and/or living conditions.[9]

It has not yet been conclusively shown whether these two approaches, one focusing more on "illness" and the other more on "health," are diametrically opposed or perhaps two sides of the same coin. More research is needed. Research among art therapists (Pénzes, 2020) shows that while art therapists pay attention to the client's challenges, symptoms, and their severity, they also pay explicit attention to the client's strengths, possibilities, and potential space for change.

In ArTA, it is assumed that mental health is not a black and white concept. A person is neither completely healthy nor completely ill. Mental health cannot be defined solely by the absence of symptoms. Even with symptoms, a person can live a healthy and meaningful life. Adversity is inherent in life. Mental health is defined by adaptability: the ability to cope with events and situations that may trigger negative thoughts and emotions. This is also known as resilience or psychological flexibility. It is important to be aware of the symptoms but to focus on the opportunities/healthy aspects that are present in order to strengthen them where possible. At the same time, it is important to make a realistic assessment of the level and type of support a client will need when adaptability is (temporarily) limited. For this reason, ArTA does not lead to the formulation of a diagnosis, but rather to the formulation of an assessment. Two concepts are important in this regard: balance and adaptability. Both are important to mental health.

Balance is the integration between thinking and feeling. The ability to recognize, allow, appropriately express, and regulate feelings through cognitive control contributes to mental health.

Adaptability is the ability to cope with and adjust to the various situations and challenges that life brings. Balance and adaptability are interrelated. They are first described separately below and then the relationship will be explained. Since art therapists focus on the client's health, it would be expected to start with adaptability. In practice, however, the client's request for help is always the reason and the beginning of the treatment. In ArTA, we look at this request for help from the concept of balance.

1.4.1 Balance

The balance between thinking and feeling is very important for mental health. Thinking is about thoughts, cognitions, and cognitive processes such as planning, organizing, analyzing, and structuring. It is not so much about the content, but the degree of cognitive control. Feeling is about sensations, feelings, and emotions and the ability to recognize, allow, and express them appropriately.

Balance exists when a client can recognize, allow, and accept feelings, even negative ones, and express them in such a way that they do not take over. In other words, a person can access their feelings and regulate them through cognitive control. Both processes – thinking and feeling – are important for balanced functioning and mental health.

In clients there is usually an imbalance. Thinking or feeling dominates and determines behavior and this can interfere with healthy functioning. When feeling dominates, clients may have difficulty regulating their emotions: they may be overwhelmed by them and feel unable to control them. If thinking dominates, clients may tend to approach things "from the head," possibly because they want to avoid feelings and/or find it difficult to allow, express, and/or accept them.

1.4.2 Adaptability

Adaptability refers to the ability to adapt to different situations and challenges in (daily) life. Observing adaptability provides insight into potential areas of development. Whereas balance indicates which patterns of thinking, feeling the client has internalized, adaptability indicates how fixed these patterns are and where there is room to move toward change. Some situations require a more cognitive approach, others a more emotional one. If someone can adapt to the situation, this shows adaptability. This has many similarities to concepts such as resilience, coping, experiential acceptance, and psychological flexibility.

A number of aspects determine adaptability: self-management, flexibility, openness, and creativity (see Figure 1.7).

Self-management has to do with the ability to make decisions and carry them out. Someone with sufficient self-management can step back, reflect, pay attention to a given situation, and act accordingly. It can be related to self-determination, identity, and autonomy. Self-management may be limited if someone has a lot of doubt and finds it difficult to pay attention to and/or implement their own preferences, ideas, and opinions.

Flexibility refers to the range of abilities to respond to a variety of challenges, tasks, people, and situations. It requires the ability to switch between thinking and feeling as appropriate. Flexibility can be limited when a person has fixed or rigid patterns of thinking, feeling, and acting. It may then be difficult to switch between different ways of responding and adapting to the situation.

Openness has to do with an attitude in which a person wants to take in different perspectives. It involves curiosity, taking risks, not seeing mistakes as catastrophic, and daring to experiment in new situations. Openness may be limited if someone has difficulty dealing with unfamiliar situations.

Creativity refers to the ability to deviate from usual habits and strategies in order to discover something new. Someone with sufficient creativity has the ability to combine things and create something new. It is related to the ability to solve problems. Creativity can be limited if someone prefers to stick to familiar ways of responding, even if they are inappropriate for a given situation or hinder their own development and health.

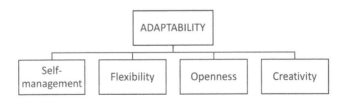

Figure 1.7 Adaptability consists of self-management, flexibility, openness, and creativity.

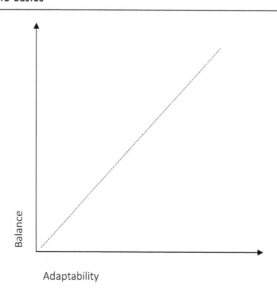

Figure 1.8 Relationship between balance and adaptability.

Self-management, flexibility, openness, and creativity are closely related. Their combination determines adaptability. By describing them separately here, we receive a more nuanced picture of the client's adaptability. In the context of observation and assessment, this can help to evaluate where possible bottlenecks are for a client and, more importantly, where there may be room to move and an entry point for further treatment. In general, clients who struggle with these aspects have less adaptability.

Adaptability is related to balance: the more balance, the more adaptability (see Figure 1.8). The more fixed the patterns of thinking or feeling, the more difficult it seems to be to switch between them. It is important to gain insight into: 1) whether a client has fixed patterns, and if so, which ones and to what extent they are disruptive or experienced as such and 2) how fixed these patterns are, in order to assess whether there is room for change. This is important for determining whether the client might benefit from art therapy and, if so, for formulating treatment goals, choosing the appropriate art interventions, and estimating the length of treatment needed (see also §2.12).

1.5 Neuroanalogous processes

Because there are different views of both art therapy and mental health, there are also different views of the relationship between the two. All these differences make it complex to study and describe the relationship between art and mental health. Some older research suggests a relationship between the art form and psychopathology (see also §2.2). More recent research shows that the art form is re-lated to both pathological and healthy aspects (e.g., Abbing, 2020; Haeyen, 2018).

Within ArTA, disease and health are considered on a continuum, and so there is always a healthy part present. In addition, it is assumed that mental health is closely related to physical health. Body and mind are one and determine healthy functioning. It assumes that our body, mind, brain, immune, and hormonal systems are all one. A person who is functioning in a healthy way is balanced (see §1.4.1) and can respond adaptively to daily and challenging situations (see §1.4.2). This involves several neurobiological and neuropsychological processes. These processes are analogous to those activated in art therapy. Hence the term neuroanalogous processes.

In ArTA, this specifically concerns the art form. Working with art materi-als in an art-making process that results in an art product is what distinguishes art therapy from other forms of therapy. Based on research (see §2.1), it has been shown that there is a clear relationship between the art form and balance and adaptability as aspects of mental health. Neuroanalogical processes refer to the similarity between the processes that influence mental health and thus drive daily functioning and the processes activated during art making. And this relationship is reciprocal. This means that aspects of mental health and daily functioning – especially balance and adaptability – become visible and tangible in art-making and the art product, but also that changes in art-making – when methodically applied by an art therapist – leads to change in mental health.

Let us first take a closer look at what neurological processes are important for health and daily functioning. And then how they are analogous to the processes activated during art-making in art therapy.

1.5.1 A neuroscientific approach to health

Daily (dis)functioning is driven by the ingenious interplay of various neuro-biological and neuropsychological processes. Many of these processes are controlled by subcortical and cortical neural networks. Cortical processes are controlled by the newer and higher parts of the brain, particularly the cortex. For example, the (pre)frontal cortex plays an important role in regulating emotions and in executive functions such as attention, concentration, reflection, meaning-making, and planning. Specifically, the middle prefrontal region is crucial for the connection with subcortical areas such as the limbic system and the brainstem (Siegel, 2011). Subcortical processes take place at an unconscious level and are controlled by the deeper parts of the brain, such as the limbic system and auto-nomic nervous system.

The limbic system, located deep in the center of the brain, is intimately in-volved with emotions, emotional memory, motivation, and pleasure (Freberg, 2018). It is constantly scanning the environment: is it safe or unsafe? In this way, the limbic system helps create emotions that urge the body to move away from the unsafe and toward the safe.

As a result, the limbic system makes an important contribution to adaptability by helping to respond appropriately to a variety of situations. The limbic system also has an important regulatory function through the hypothalamus, a central control center for the endocrine system. For example, in unsafe, stressful situations, the so-called hypothalamic-pituitary-adrenal (HPA) axis produces cortisol, which mobilizes the body to fight or flight. This is adaptive. The limbic system also helps create emotional memory. In particular, the amygdala and the hippocampus that are part of the limbic system play a role in this. For example, the amygdala activates a fear response, activating the HPA-axis and sympathetic nervous system (see below). This happens very fast, even without the intervention of the expanded consciousness. This allows a very quick response to threatening situations and thus helps survival. LeDoux (1998) called this the speedy low road. In parallel, the same stimulus that activated the amygdala goes to the cortex, where a more conscious meaning is given to the stimulus. LeDoux called this the thinking high road. This can lead to the stimulus being interpreted as safe and the amygdala being inhibited. The body then recovers from the stress and restores balance, which is highly adaptive. This also shows how the subcortical limbic system is connected to the cortex and to the brainstem, which, in turn, is closely connected to the autonomic nervous system.

The primary functions of the autonomic nervous system are survival and homeostasis. The autonomic nervous system consists of the sympathetic nervous system, which is activated when danger is perceived, and the parasympathetic nervous system, which contributes to rest and recovery. A properly functioning autonomic nervous system is therefore balanced and adaptive. The autonomic nervous system controls all the automatic functions in the body, such as breathing, digestion, heart rate, etc. Think of it as a "cruise control." These processes are responses to stimuli from the body, such as hunger and sleep, and stimuli from the environment. Being able to adequately signal stimuli of safety and unsafety helps the body respond adaptively and thus survive. When the body signals danger, the sympathetic nervous system is activated: the heart rate increases, breathing accelerates, and cortisol and adrenaline are produced. In short, the body prepares to mobilize. When the body signals safety the parasympathetic nervous system is activated: the body returns to rest and recovers. In this way, a healthy autonomic nervous system is balanced and adaptive.

In addition, the autonomic nervous system plays an important role in integration with other subcortical and cortical processes. This is because the autonomic nervous system is connected to all the organs in our body and to other subcortical and cortical brain structures. For example, the amygdala activates and deactivates the hormonal and immune systems. But also cortical processes such as the regulatory effect of the (pre-) frontal cortex, which plays an important role in executive functions such as attention, concentration, and planning. The regulation and integration of these different networks is important for healthy and balanced functioning. This allows to respond adaptively to everyday and challenging situations, to become aware of, express and regulate inner experiences and feelings. Becoming aware of feelings helps to regulate these emotions and creates space for understanding and compassion for one's own physical and emotional reaction, on the one hand, and for responding differently, on the other. Thus, integration of different subcortical and cortical processes is of great importance for balance and adaptability.

The involved networks are anatomically more or less the same in everyone. However, research (Cozolino, 2017; Perry & Ablon, 2019; Porges, 2003, 2017; Siegel, 2010, 2012, 2019, 2020; Van der Kolk et al., 2012) shows that their programming, in addition to genes, is largely dependent on acquired experiences. This is certainly the case for the subcortical processes that are controlled by the limbic system and the autonomic nervous system. And these processes largely determine our behavior (Cozolino, 2017; Damasio, 2003, 2010, 2021; Greenberg, 2002; Hayes et al., 1999; Kahneman, 2011; LeDoux, 1998; Porges, 2003, 2017; Siegel, 2010, 2012, 2020; Stern, 2000, 2010; Van der Kolk, 2014; Van der Kolk et al., 2012). This means that these processes take place at an unconsciousness level and that much of our behavior is controlled automatically, without our continuous extended thought and awareness.

Experiences that are challenging but manageable contribute to the development of adaptability. Experiences that are uncontrollable, unpredictable, or unmanageable, such as trauma and chronic stress, disrupt the processes that are so important for physical and mental health. They become dysregulated, fragmented, and unbalanced. Feeling or thinking then take over and people become stuck in unconscious and often rigid patterns of thinking, feeling, and acting. This may result in a variety of physical and psychological ailments. This is often the case with clients. They experience imbalance and (temporarily) lack adaptability. Because experiences vary from person to person, ArTA places great value on the uniqueness of each client. And while we can make statements about patterns of balance and adaptability based on systematic observation of material interaction, material experience, and the art product, the color of those statements will vary from person to person. As these processes are mainly developed through acquired experiences, they are difficult to influence (only) through cognition and language, but mainly through purposeful new experiences. That's where art therapy comes in.

1.5.2 Analogies between neurological processes and art-making

Analogous processes are known within the context of arts therapies primarily from Smeijsters' analogue process model (Smeijsters, 2008, 2012). This model is based on the work of Damasio (2003), Greenberg (2002), LeDoux (1998), and Stern (2000), among others. The basic idea is that the processes that are activated during art therapy are analogous to the processes that determine health and thus daily functioning. Based on insights from recent neuroscientific research in the field of art and art therapy, this theory has been updated in the context of ArTA.

Neuroscience research has gained tremendous momentum in recent years, in part, due to the increase in technical research possibilities, for example, (f)MRI and EEG. Research at the intersection of art – neuroaesthetics – and art therapy is increasing. It is beyond the scope of this book to give a complete overview.[10]

Neuroscience is still a relatively young branch of research, especially in the field of art therapy. Undoubtedly, more knowledge will be gained in the (near) future. Nevertheless, it is interesting to see how current findings contribute to an understanding of how and why art-making in art therapy is related to mental health. Based on this research, three aspects of art therapy that are relevant to the rationale of ArTA are highlighted. These aspects include (1) the importance of experience, (2) the importance of movement, and (3) the integrative effect of art-making.

1.5.2.1 The importance of experience

Section 1.5.1 described how the interplay of various cortical and subcortical processes affects daily functioning. Integration of these processes is very important for healthy functioning. Otherwise, fragmentation and dysregulation occur. This disrupts balance (see §1.4.1) and limits adaptability (see §1.4.2). It has also been described that subcortical processes in particular largely control behavior and are developed on the basis of experience. Also, subcortical processes occur at a subconscious, noncognitive level. Therefore, these processes are less easily influenced by cognition or language, but rather by the acquisition of specific new experiences.

Art-making in art therapy also takes place at an subconscious, noncognitive level, is action-oriented and explicitly experiential. Therefore, it provides a good entry point for influencing the processes described above and for initiating change. Because art-making in art therapy appeals primarily to doing, especially by interacting with art materials cognition and words are not initially involved, and immediate experiences in the here and now arise (Hass-Cohen & Carr, 2008; Hass-Cohen & Findlay, 2015; Hass-Cohen et al., 2018; Stern, 2010).

The different properties of the art materials (see §1.3) have different experiential qualities.[11] By methodically using the properties of these materials, in combination with techniques and instructions (see §1.3), the client arrives at a different way of structuring the art-making and acquires different experiences. These experiences can be placed on a continuum from cognitive to affective (see Table 1.1). This is a continuum because of the wide variety of possible combinations of materials, techniques, tools, and instruction.

Cognitive experiences occur when the art-making process is structured in such a way that the client is encouraged to think for themselves about what is

Table 1.1 How combinations of materials, techniques and tools, and instructions affect the art-making experience

Cognitive experience		Affective experience
Materials	Solid materials such as pencils, markers, and crayons that provide good grip and are easy to control.	Fluid materials that invite experimentation, such as watercolor and sensory materials like finger paint.
Techniques and tools	Linear techniques, such as drawing and coloring and techniques that involve many steps, such as lino printing.	Pictorial techniques such as blending/mixing, washing out and flowing.
Instructions	Low level of instruction (lots of choice) with high complexity (specific outcome required).	Some degree of instruction (provides clarity) and limited degree of complexity (no specific outcome required).

being made and how it can be done. Working systematically toward a specific result is usually central. Instruction plays an important role here, especially low-level (low degree and low complexity) instructions that give a lot of freedom of choice and actively encourage the client to think for themselves (as opposed to high-level instructions where everything is already determined). Materials and techniques also play an important role. Solid materials tend to provide more support and are easier to control than fluid materials. Techniques that involve many steps and/or a fixed sequence, such as making a linoleum print, activate more cognition than a coincidental technique. Similarly, more linear techniques, such as drawing, activate more cognition than pictorial techniques, such as painting.

Affective experiences occur when the art-making process is structured to activate the client to feel the material and to experience what is being made and how it is being made. Trying out the material and experimenting with the possibilities without a specific result is usually central to this. A limited amount of instruction (some complexity and degree of instruction) contributes to this. Some level and complexity of instruction, possibly focused on experimentation and feeling, encourages the client to feel; the client has clarity and does not have to think for themselves. Low level and low complexity of instruction provides a lot of freedom of choice and is more likely to lead the client to cognition. High complexity leaves little room for feeling, as the client must remember and perform many steps. Fluid materials tend to have more application possibilities, are more inviting to play and experiment with, and contribute to an affective experience (Corem et al., 2015; Hinz, 2020; Pénzes et al., 2014, 2015; Regev & Snir, 2018;

Snir & Regev, 2013a, 2013b). Materials that require direct physical contact (also called sensory materials), such as finger paint, contribute by their sensation to an affective experience (Haiblum-Itskovitch et al., 2018; Hinz, 2020; Hyland Moon, 2010; Malchiodi, 2012; Naff, 2014; Pénzes, 2020; Pénzes et al., 2023; Rubin, 2009; Regev & Snir, 2018; Snir & Regev, 2013a).

Dysregulation, fragmentation, and imbalance can manifest in a variety of ways. When feelings predominate, functioning may be strongly determined by subcortical processes. For example, someone who has experienced trauma may have difficulty feeling safe. Signals are quickly and sometimes unnecessarily perceived as unsafe, so the sympathetic nervous system is always "on," ready to mobilize in response to the perceived stimulus of insecurity and stress. Because a person subconsciously does not experience a sense of safety, the parasympathetic nervous system is no longer activated, preventing rest and recovery. In addition, a sense of safety is necessary to connect with one's body and emotions. The remarkable thing about emotions is that we can't distinguish between avoiding negative and positive emotions: if we unconsciously avoid negative emotions, we also deprive ourselves of experiencing positive emotions such as joy and play. Because of this dysregulation, a person becomes unconsciously stuck in rigid patterns characterized by feelings of anxiety, depression, or emotional flattening where there is no room for curiosity and exploration of possibilities. Art therapy can provide a safe context in which to play, relax, and experience success. It can provide space to become aware of body signals and feelings and to acknowledge them rather than avoid them. It can provide space to experience that emotions are always temporary and that negative emotions such as sadness and fear will pass. This allows the client to experience that emotions can be tolerated as well as expressed and redirected. This contributes to a sense of self, creating space for exploration of new experiences that may not have immediate expression in words.

In order for the client to have specific experiences in art therapy that contribute to the treatment process, it is important to gain insight into how the client structures the art-making process, what preferences the client has for materials and techniques, how the client interacts with the material, and how the client experiences the material. We saw in Section 1.4 that healthy functioning is balanced and adaptive. Clients usually have an imbalance between thinking and feeling and it is important to gain insight into this. Does the client tend to think more or feel more? To what extent? And how does this limit the adaptability? The systematic observation of these aspects helps the art therapist to assess whether the client could benefit from art therapy. This is called an indication.[12] This immediately underscores the importance of a thorough art therapy assessment: it is crucial for formulating treatment goals and selecting art therapy interventions that will actually enable the client to have experiences that will enable them to work on treatment goals and engage in a process of change.

1.5.2.2 The importance of movement

The subcortical processes that play such an important role in healthy functioning take place at a subconscious, noncognitive level and are therefore expressed less in language and more in movement. Damasio (2010, 2021) introduces the concept of "core self" which is relevant in this context. The core self is a felt, intuitive, noncognitive form of knowing, based on acquired experiences. As a result, people instinctively "know" what is going on inside them and how they react to the outside world, even if they cannot explain it in words and concepts. This "felt knowing" is anchored in the body and expressed through what Stern (2010) calls vitality forms. Vitality forms are feeling processes that take place in the inner self and are expressed in a particular time sequence and form through a combination of parameters such as tempo, rhythm, number, intensity, movement, and form. Examples of vitality forms are vigorous, calm, energetic, rushing, collapsing, slowing down, and so on. This also means that dysregulation and fragmentation, leading to imbalance and limited adaptability, become visible in movement.

For example, a person experiencing chronic stress may feel overwhelmed. The situations are unpredictable or unmanageable. This affects the sense of self and sense of agency and may lead to hyperarousal. A person may feel continuously rushed and agitated and is in a constant state of readiness to respond to the stressful situation. This is reflected in movement that is, for example, rushed, tense of erratic.

Art therapy, by definition, is action-oriented. Movement drives and becomes visible in the art-making process, specifically in material interaction (see §2.4). For example, the person above experiencing hyperarousal, whose movement is characterized by high speed, volatility, and tension will interact with the art materials in a different way than someone who is relaxed and in control of the situation. This, in turn, becomes manifest in the formal elements of the art product, especially its movement, dynamic, and contour (see §2.6.1). These express the forms of vitality that are so characteristic of the client's functioning. Observing patterns in material interaction, material experience, and the art product provides insight into how clients deal with challenges and other situations outside of therapy. It also indicates the client's ability to explore emotions and thoughts (balance) and additionally the extent to which the client can experiment with other coping strategies and create new solutions (adaptability). And because movement is closely related to emotion, it is also tangible, specifically in the material experience (see §2.5). So the processes activated in art therapy are analogous to the processes that drive functioning outside of therapy.

And that's good news, because it also means that when you allow someone to move in a different way, to interact with art materials in a different way, you are influencing those processes and working toward change. By initiating a different directed movement, accompanied by a different directed experience, a person can experience "first hand" what it does. The art therapist is uniquely qualified to use the art form methodically in this process and to tailor it specifically to the client. Especially to the client's strength. Through constructive art-making, this healthy part is addressed and the client comes to a different way of structuring the art-making and thus gains different experiences. For example, through (controlled) mobilization or just relaxation, sensing how the body responds to sensory stimuli (e.g., in interaction with the art material), perceiving what emotion is associated with it, and how that emotion can be felt, tolerated, and expressed in a safe context. This increases the sense of self and agency, restores the balance between thinking and feeling, and contributes to adaptability.

Again, it is important to stress the importance of a good art therapy assessment. By using ArTA to get a good sense of the direction and degree of imbalance and aspects of adaptability, the art form can be tailored to restore the client's balance between feeling and thinking and increase adaptability. Literally and figuratively, this gets the client moving toward health.

1.5.2.3 The integrating effect of art-making

We have already seen in §1.5.1 that there is usually a disintegration in clients: the subcortical and cortical processes are fragmented. As a result, thinking or feeling takes over. For example, it's difficult for clients whose functioning is dominated by thinking, driven by cortical processes, to become aware of their own bodies and feelings. Cognitive control is then paramount, which can lead to overuse of cognition. In contrast, clients whose functioning is dominated by feeling, driven by subcortical processes, may find it difficult to regulate or adequately express their feelings.

For example, a client who was overwhelmed by an experience while making art may benefit from stepping back from the experience. By reflecting with the therapist, the client gains insight into what happened and why. A pattern of possible triggers may also emerge, possibly across sessions. By being aware of this, the client may be able to recognize it more easily and earlier so that the feelings do not take over so easily in the future.

An art-making process requires not only doing and experiencing but also cognition. Allowing the experience during art-making to be there and reflecting on it (together with the therapist) activates cortical processes and contributes to the client's awareness. In an art-making process, one can work form sensing to perception to awareness. This can be attuned to the client's need and ability to reflect (see §2.10). By taking distance from the art-making and the experience, clients become aware of patterns in their own functioning, within and outside the therapy, and can assign a different meaning to them. By working in the here and now, the client is given the opportunity to experience that patterns of functioning that were helpful or even necessary in the past are no longer functional.

This contributes to understanding of and self-compassion for rigid pattern in daily functioning. Understanding that they are not stuck in these patterns that are no longer functional, adds meaning and helps redirect negative thoughts and feelings and do things differently than before. This creates space to take more or different perspectives and explore different ways of responding, leading a more balanced and adaptive functioning within the client's capacity.

Notes

1 'Analogous processes' are known within the context of arts therapies primarily from Smeijsters' analogue process model. This model finds its basis in the work of Damasio (2003), Greenberg (2002), LeDoux (1998) and Stern (2000), among others. Based on insights from recent neuroscience research in the field of art therapy, this theory has been updated in the context of ArTA (see §1.5).

2 There are several review articles available. I find the article by Van Lith (2016) very clear. The various (international) professional associations also provide definitions of art therapy such as the American Art Therapy Association [AATA] (n.d.), the British Association of Art Therapists [BAAT] (n.d.) and the Dutch Association for Art Therapy [Nederlandse Vereniging voor Beeldende Therapie: NVBT] (n.d.).

3 The art form as a distinctive aspect of art therapy may be taken for granted in practice and literature. Some sources: Edwards (2013), Hinz (2020), Hyland Moon (2010), Jue and Hee Ha (2021) and McNiff (2019).

4 It is not only within ArTA that this is being addressed. Previous authors also wrote about it including Beerse et al. (2020) and Lorenzo de la Pena (2016).

5 Much has traditionally been written about this within art therapy: including Betensky (2001), Haiblum-Itskovitch et al. (2018), Hinz (2020), Hyland Moon (2010), Kagin and Lusebrink (1978), Kramer (1971), Regev and Snir (2018), Rhyne (1973), Pénzes et al. (2014, 2015), Pesso-Aviv et al. (2014) and Snir and Regev (2013a).

6 This is not yet about the experience this may evoke in a client. One client may like this (for example, if a client is skilled in drawing by observation and/or enjoys doing this), another client may find this exciting or even frustrating (for example, if the client sets the bar very high, but lacks the skill). We will return to this later in Section 2.4 on material experience.

7 This way of describing instruction comes originally from Hinz's Expressive Therapies Continuum [ETC] (2020). In the "Creative Minds" research project, we investigated how instruction affects brain activity (Pénzes et al., 2023).

8 Much has been written criticizing such classification systems. I find the views of Van der Kolk et al. (2012), Van der Kolk (2014), Van Os et al. (2019) and Veereschild et al. (2020) worth reading.

9 Relatively much is written about the critique of the so-called positive health for vulnerable groups. A clear study I find to be that of Rössler (2018).

10 Some interesting sources are Czamanski-Cohen and Weihs (2016), Hass-Cohen et al. (2018), Hinz (2020), Kaimal et al. (2016), Kaimal et al. (2018), King (2016), King and Kaimal (2019), King et al. (2017), King et al. (2019), King and Parada (2021), Magsamen and Ross (2023), Payano Sosa et al. (2023) and Pénzes et al. (2023).

11 There has traditionally been much attention within art therapy to experiential qualities, or as in ArTA called material experience (Betensky, 1973, 2001; Hass-Cohen & Carr, 2008; Hass-Cohen & Findlay, 2015; Hinz, 2020; Hyland Moon, 2010; Kramer,

1975; Lusebrink, 1990, 2010; Malchiodi, 2012; Rhyne, 1973; Rubin, 2005, 2009, 2011; Schnetz, 2005; Seiden, 2001; Virshup et al., 1993).

12 Indication refers to the recommendation for further treatment. Within ArTA, indication is positioned as part of assessment. One cannot exist without the other (see Section 2.11).

References

Abbing, A.C. (2020). *Art therapy & anxiety* [Doctoral dissertation, Leiden University]. Retrieved from https://hdl.handle.net/1887/83276

American Art Therapy Association [AATA]. (n.d.). *About art therapy.* Consulted on July 9, 2023 on https://arttherapy.org/about-art-therapy/

American Psychiatric Association [APA]. (2013). *Diagnostic and statistical manual of mental disorders* (5th ed.). https://doi.org/10.1176/appi.books.9780890425596

Antonovsky, A. (1979). *Health, stress and coping.* Jossey-Bass.

Beerse, M.E., Van Lith, T., & Standwood, G. (2020). Therapeutic psychological and biological responses to mindfulness-based art therapy. *Stress & Health, 36*(4), 419–432. https://doi.org/10.1002/smi.2937

Betensky, M.G. (1973). *Self-discovery through self-expression: Use of art psychotherapy with and adolescents.* Charles C. Thomas.

Betensky, M.G. (2001). Phenomenological art therapy. In J.A. Rubin (Ed.), *Approaches to art therapy* (2nd ed., pp. 121–133). Brunner-Routledge.

British Association of Art Therapists [BAAT]. (n.d.). *About art therapy.* Consulted on July 9, 2023 on https://www.baat.org/About-BAAT

Corem, S., Snir, S., & Regev, D. (2015). Patients' attachment to therapists in art therapy simulation and their reactions to the experience of using art materials. *The Arts in Psychotherapy, 45*, 11–17. https://doi.org/10.1016/j.aip.2015.04.006

Cozolino, L. (2017). *The neuroscience of psychotherapy, healing the social brain.* W.W.Norton & Company.

Czamanski-Cohen, J., & Weihs, K.L. (2016). The bodymind model: A platform for studying the mechanisms of change induced by art therapy. *The Arts in Psychotherapy, 51*, 63–71. https://doi.org/10.1016/j.aip.2016.08.006

Damasio, A.R. (2003). *Ik voel dus ik ben. Hoe gevoel en lichaam ons bewustzijn vormen* [I feel therefore I am. How feeling and body form our consciousness]. Wereldbibliotheek.

Damasio, A.R. (2010). *De vergissing van Descartes. Gevoel verstand en het menselijk brein [Descartes' error. Emotion, reason and the human brain].* Wereldbibliotheek.

Damasio. (2021). *Feeling & knowing. Making minds conscious.* Pantheon.

Dutch Association for Art Therapy [Nederlandse Vereniging voor Beeldende Therapie, NVBT]. (n.d.). *Beeldende therapie maakt het zichtbaar [Art therapy makes it visible].* Consulted on July 9, 2023 on: https://nvbt.vaktherapie.nl/cli%C3%ABnten-en-verwijzers

Edwards, D. (2013). *Art therapy. Creative therapies in practice* (2nd ed.). Sage.

Freberg, L.A. (2018). *Discovering behavioral neuroscience. An introduction to biological psychology* (4th ed.) Cengage.

Greenberg, L.S. (2002). *Emotion-focused therapy. Coaching clients to work through their feelings.* American Psychological Association.

Haeyen, S. (2018). *Effects of art therapy. The case of personality disorders cluster B/C* [PhD dissertation, Radboud University Nijmegen]. Behavioural Science Institute. 183225.pdf (ru.nl)

Haiblum-Itskovitch, S., Czamanski-Cohen, J., & Galili, G. (2018). Emotional response and changes in heart rate variability following art-making with three different art materials. *Frontiers in Psychology*. https://doi.org/10.3389/fpsyg.2018.00968

Hass-Cohen, N., Bokoch, R., Findlay, J., & Banford-Witting, A. (2018). A four-drawing art therapy, trauma and resiliency protocol study. *The Arts in Psychotherapy, 61*, 44–56. https://doi.org/10.1016/j.aip.2018.02.003ar

Hass-Cohen, N., & Carr, R. (2008). *Art therapy and clinical neuroscience*. Jessica Kingsley.

Hass-Cohen, N., & Findlay, J.D. (2015). *Art therapy and the neuroscience of relationships, creativity and resiliency: Skills and practices*. W.W. Norton.

Hayes, S.C., Strosahl, K.D., & Wilson, K.G. (1999). *Acceptance and commitment therapy: An experiential approach to behavior change*. The Guilford Press.

Hinz, L.D. (2020). *Expressive therapies continuum: A framework for using art in therapy* (2nd ed.). Routledge Taylor & Francis.

Huber, M., van Vliet, M., Giezenberg, M., Winkens, B., Heerkens, Y., Dagnelie, P.C., & Knottnerus, J.A. (2016). Towards a 'patient-centered' operationalisation of the new dynamic concept of health: a mixed methods study. *BMJ Open*. 2016;6:e010091. https://bmjopen.bmj.com/content/bmjopen/6/1/e010091.full.pdf

Hyland Moon, C. (2010). *Materials and media in Art Therapy*. Routledge.

Jue, J., & Hee Ha, J. (2021). Influence of art therapy students' art practice on their professional identity and career commitment. *Art Therapy: Journal of the American Art Therapy Association, 38*(1), 13–21. https://doi.org/10.1080/07421656.2020.1743609

Kagin, S.L., & Lusebrink, V.B. (1978). The expressive therapies continuum. *Art Psychotherapy, 5*, 171–180.

Kahneman, D. (2011). *Thinking, fast and slow*. Farrar, Straus and Giroux.

Kaimal, G., Ray, K., & Muniz, J.M. (2016). Reduction of cortisol levels and participants' responses following artmaking. *Art Therapy. Journal of the American Art Therapy Association, 33*(2), 74–80. doi:10.1080/07421656.2016.1166832

Kaimal, G., Walker, M.S., Herres, J., French, L.M., & DeGraba, T.J. (2018). Observational study of associations between visual imagery and measures of depression, anxiety and post-traumatic stress among active-duty military service members with traumatic brain injury at the Walter Reed National Military Medical Center. *BMJ Open, 8*(6), e021448. doi:10.1136/bmjopen-2017-021448

King, J.L. (2016). *Art therapy, trauma, and neuroscience: Theoretical and practical perspectives* (1st ed.). Routledge.

King, J.L., & Kaimal, G. (2019). Approaches to research in art therapy using imaging technologies. *Frontiers in Human Neuroscience*. https://doi.org/10.3389/fnhum.2019.00159

King, J.L., Kaimal, G., Konopka, L., Belkofer, C., & Strang, C.E. (2019). Practical applications of neuroscience-informed art therapy. *Art Therapy: Journal of the American Art Therapy Association, 36*(3), 149–156. https://doi.org/10.1080/07421656.201 9.1649549

King, J.L., Knapp, K.E., Shaikh, A., Li, F., Sabau, D., Pascuzzi, R.M., et al. (2017). Cortical activity changes after art making and rote motor movement as measured by EEG: A preliminary study. *Biomedical Journal of Scientific & Technical Research, 1*, 1–21. https://doi.org/10.26717/BJSTR.2017.01.000366

King, J.L., & Parada, F.J. (2021). Using mobile brain/body imaging to advance research in arts, health, and related therapeutics. *European Journal of Neuroscience, 54*, 8364–8380. https://doi.org/10.1111/ejn.15313

Knottnerus, J.A. (2016). Towards a 'patient-centered' operationalisation of the new dynamic concept of health: A mixed methods study. *BMJ Open, 6,* e010091. https://bmjopen.bmj.com/content/bmjopen/6/1/e010091.full.pdf

Kramer, E. (1971). *Art as therapy with children.* Schocken.

Kramer, E. (1975). The problem of quality in art. In E. Ulman & P. Dachinger (Eds.), *Art therapy in theory and practice* (pp. 43–59). Schocken.

LeDoux, J. (1998). *The emotional brain: The mysterious underpinnings of emotional life.* Touchstone.

Lorenzo de la Pena, S. (2016). 2D expression is intrinsic. In D.E. Gussak & M.L. Rosal (Eds.), *The Wiley handbook of art therapy.* John Wiley & Sons.

Lusebrink, V.B. (1990). *Imagery and visual expression in therapy.* Plenum.

Lusebrink, V.B. (2010). Assessment and therapeutic application of the expressive therapies continuum: Implication for brain structures and functions. *Art Therapy: Journal of the American Art Therapy Association, 27*(4), 168–177. https://doi.org/10.1080/07421656.2010.10129380

Magsamen, S., & Ross, I. (2023). *Your brain on art. How the arts transform us.* Canongate.

Malchiodi, C.A. (2012). *Handbook of art therapy.* The Guilford Press.

McNiff, S. (2019). Reflections on what "art" does in art therapy practice and research. *Art Therapy: Journal of the American Art Therapy Association, 36*(3), 162–165. https://doi.org//10.1080/07421656.2019.1649547

Naff, K. (2014). A framework for treating cumulative trauma with art therapy. *Art Therapy Journal of the American Art Therapy Association, 31*(2), 79–86. https://doi.org/10.1080/07421656.2014.903824

Payano Sosa, J., Srikanchana, R., Walker, M., Stamper, A., King, J.L., Ollinger, J., Bonavia, G., Workman, C., Darda, K., Chatterjee, A., & Sours Rhodes, C. (2023). Increased functional connectivity in military service members presenting a psychological closure and healing theme in art therapy masks. *The Arts in Psychotherapy, 85.* https://doi.org/10.1016/j.aip.2023.102050

Pénzes, I. (2020). *Art form and mental health. Studies on art therapy observation and assessment in adult mental health* [PhD dissertation, Radboud University Nijmegen]. Behavioral Science Institute. https://repository.ubn.ru.nl/bitstream/handle/2066/216188/216188.pdf?sequence=1

Pénzes, I., Engelbert, R., Heidendael, D., Oti, K., Jongen, E.M.M., & Van Hooren, S. (2023). The influence of art material and instruction during art making on brain activity: A quantitative electroencephalogram study. *The Arts in Psychotherapy, 83.* https://doi.org/10.1016/j.aip.2023.102024

Pénzes, I., van Hooren, S., Dokter, D., Smeijsters, H., & Hutschemaekers, G. (2014). Material interaction in art therapy assessment. *The Arts in Psychotherapy, 41,* 484–492. https://doi.org/10.1016/j.aip.2014.08.003

Pénzes, I., van Hooren, S., Dokter, D., Smeijsters, H., & Hutschemaekers, G. (2015). Material interaction and art product in art therapy assessment in adult mental health. *Arts & Health, 8*(3), 213–228. https://doi.org/10.1080/17533015.2015.1088557

Perry, B.D., & Ablon, J.S. (2019). CPS as a neurodevelopmentally sensitive and trauma-informed approach. In A. Pollastri, J. Ablon, & M. Hone (Eds.), *Collaborative problem solving. Current clinical psychiatry.* Springer. https://doi.org/10.1007/978-3-030-12630-8_2

Pesso-Aviv, T., Regev, D., & Guttmann, J. (2014). The unique therapeutic effect of different art materials on psychological aspects of 7- to 9-year-old children. *The Arts in Psychotherapy, 41*, 293–301. https://doi.org/10.1016/j.aip.2014.04.005

Porges, S.W. (2003). The polyvagal theory: Phylogenetic contributions to social behavior. *Physiology & Behavior, 79*, 503–513. https://doi.org/10.1016/S0031-9384(03)00156-2

Porges, S.W. (2017). *The pocket guide to the polyvagal theory: The transformative power of feeling safe*. WW Norton.

Regev, D., & Snir, D. (2018). *Parent-child art psychotherapy*. Taylor & Francis.

Rhyne, J. (1973). *The Gestalt art therapy experience*. Brooks/Cole.

Rössler, B. (2018). Autonomie. *Een essay over het vervulde leven* [*Autonomy. An essay on the fulfilled life*]. Boom.

Rubin, J.A. (2005). *Artful therapy*. John Wiley & Sons.

Rubin, J.A. (2009). *Introduction to art therapy. Sources and resources*. Routledge Taylor Francis.

Rubin, J.A. (2011). *The art of art therapy: What every art therapist needs to know*. Routledge Taylor Francis.

Schnetz, M. (2005). *The healing flow: Artistic expression in therapy*. Jessica Kingsley.

Seiden, D. (2001). *Mind over matter: The uses of materials in art, education and therapy*. Magnolia Street.

Siegel, D.J. (2010). *Mind sight. Transform your brain with the new science of kindness*. OneWorld.

Siegel, D.J. (2011). *Mindsight. The new science of personal transformation*. Bentam Books.

Siegel, D.J. (2012). *The developing mind. How relationships and the brain interact to shape who we are*. The Guilford Press.

Siegel, D.J. (2019). The mind in psychotherapy: An interpersonal neurobiology framework for understanding and cultivating mental health. *Psychology and Psychotherapy: Theory, Research and Practice, 92*, 224–237. https://doi.org/10.1111/papt.12228

Siegel, D.J. (2020). *The developing mind: How relationships and the brain interact to shape who we are* (3rd ed.). The Guilford Press.

Smeijsters, H. (2012). Analogy and metaphor in music therapy. Theory and practice. *Nordic Journal of Music Therapy, 21*(3), 227–249. https://doi.org/10.1080/08098131.2011.649299

Smeijsters, H. (2008). *Handboek creatieve therapie* [*Handbook creative therapies*]. Coutinho.

Snir, S., & Regev, D. (2013a). A dialog with five art materials: Creators share their art making experiences. *The Arts in Psychotherapy, 40*(1), 94–100. https://doi.org/10.1016/j.aip.2012.11.004

Snir, S., & Regev, D. (2013b). ABI – arts-based intervention questionnaire. *The Arts in Psychotherapy, 40*(3), 94–100. https://doi.org/10.1016/j.aip.2012.11.004.

Stern, D.N. (2000). *The interpersonal world of the infant. A view from psychoanalysis and development psychology*. Basic Books.

Stern, D.N. (2010). *Forms of vitality. Exploring dynamic experience in psychology, the arts, psychotherapy, and development*. Oxford University.

Van der Kolk, B. (2014). *The body keeps the score*. Penguin.

Van der Kolk, B., McFarlane, A.C., & Weisaeth, L. (2012). *Traumatic stress. The effects of overwhelming experiences on mind body and society*. The Guilford Press.

Van Heycop ten Ham, B., Hulsbergen, M., & Bohlmeijer, E. (2014). *Transdiagnostische factoren. Theorie & Praktijk* [*Transdiagnostic factors. Theory & practice*]. Boom.

Van Lith, T. (2016). Art therapy in mental health: A systematic review of approaches and practices. *The Arts in psychotherapy, 47*(2), 9–22. http://dx.doi.org/10.1016/j.aip.2015.09.003

Van Os, J., Guloksuz, S., Vijn, T.W., Hafkenscheid, A., & Delespaul, P. (2019). The evidence-based group-level symptom-reduction model as the organizing principle for mental health care: time for change? *World Psychiatry, 18*(1), 88–96. https://doi.org/10.1002/wps.20609

Veereschild, H.M., Noorthoorn, E.O., Nijman, H.L.I., Mulder, C.L., Dankers, M., Van der Veen, J.A., Loonen, A.J.M., & Hutschemaeker, G.J.M. (2020). Diagnose, indicate, and treat severe mental illness (DITSMI) as appropriate care: A three-year follow-up study in long-term residential psychiatric patients on the effects of re-diagnosis on medication prescription, patient functioning, and hospital bed utilization. *European Psychiatry, 63*(1), 1–8. https://doi.org/10.1192/j.eurpsy.2020.46

Virshup, E., Riley, S., & Sheperd, D. (1993). The art of healing trauma: Media, techniques, and insights. In E. Virshup (Ed.), *California art therapy trends*. Magnolia Street, 429–431.

World Health Organization [WHO]. (2021). *Definition of health*. Consulted on July 9, 2023 on: https://www.publichealth.com.ng/world-health-organizationwho-definition-of-health/who-definition-of-health-2/

Chapter 2

ArTA

The theory

Introduction

Observation and assessment are often mentioned in the same breath. However, there is a difference between the two. Observation is about perception, whereas assessment is about interpreting. In the context of art therapy, observation is the focused and systematic perception of how the client shapes the art-making process and the art product. Assessment is the step of giving meaning to these observations. This means that the observations are interpreted in terms of mental health. Gaining insight into these aspects helps the art therapist to evaluate whether the client could benefit from art therapy. This is called an indication.

In Chapter 1, ArTA's vision of mental health and the importance of the art form was described. But how exactly do you know what to observe in art therapy? And how precisely can you then interpret this in terms of the client's mental health?

Several methods of art therapy observation and assessment have been developed internationally. These are based on different theoretical principles. Some methods are based on psychoanalytic, developmental, or behavioral theories. Other methods are based on art theories. Still others are eclectic. In addition, many of the methods developed are based on the clinical experience of an art therapist and have not been scientifically researched. Those methods that have been researched do not always prove to be reliable and valid.

ArTA is the first method using the evidence-based relationship between the art form and mental health. This chapter therefore begins with a summary of this research. Art therapists from different countries and with different clinical experiences and theoretical backgrounds participated in this research. By focusing on commonalities rather than differences, ArTA transcends different approaches and methods. This makes ArTA useful for all art therapists, regardless of their perspective and theoretical background.

We will then take a closer look at the methodology underlying ArTA. This includes the material interaction, the material experience, and the art product and

DOI: 10.4324/9781003428305-2

their relationship to mental health. We will also look at the role of reflection and instruction within ArTA and the indication for further treatment.

2.1   The evidence base of ArTA

ArTA is based on my doctoral research[1] and therefore evidence-based.

The primary reason for undertaking this research was to test the fundamental assumption of art therapy, namely, the assumed relationship between the art form and adult mental health. The literature at that point revealed several theoretical perspectives and rationales on the subject. There were different views on how exactly mental health is represented in the art form. They varied in the use of art materials and how they interpreted the art-making process and the art product in terms of mental health (see also §2.2).

In this research, I wanted to know (1) how art therapists with different theoretical perspectives observe the art form in art therapy assessment; (2) the art therapists' views on adult clients' mental health; and (3) whether there is a relationship between the art form and adult mental health and, if so, whether the art-making process, the art product, or both are related to specific aspects of adult clients' mental health. I examined these questions with four studies and seven sub studies using a mixed method design.

In the first qualitative study, using grounded theory methodology, I explored how art therapists with different training backgrounds and perspectives on art therapy used, observed, and interpreted the art form in assessing the mental health of adult clients. Despite their different backgrounds, the art therapists systematically used the different properties of (primarily two-dimensional) art materials – specifically their degree of physical contact, intrinsic structure, and range of technical possibilities. The art therapists observed the client's:

1 Material interaction: how the clients interacted with these properties of the art materials (see §2.4).
2 Material experience: how the clients experienced the art materials (see §2.5).
3 Art product: what clients made (see §2.6).

In the second qualitative study, using focus group methodology, I included a larger number of art therapists to further explore and theorize the concept of material interaction and its relationship to the art product and adult clients' mental health. Further examination of the initial categories of material interaction led to 12 categories which were found to be important to observe (see §2.4, Table 2.2). Dialogue was considered a core concept as it connected all the other categories. Because the categories of material interaction were strongly interrelated, their combination formed a material interaction style that could be placed on a continuum from rational to affective. A rational style of material interaction often indicated a client's tendency to cognitive control. Clients with a tendency to control were often considered to be very thoughtful, precise, and perfectionistic, and to have difficulty recognizing, experiencing, and expressing emotions, or to try to avoid them (see §2.4.1). Clients who exhibited an affective style of material interaction could be easily overwhelmed by emotions, have difficulty regulating emotions and structuring their impulses, and may have difficulty with boundaries (see §2.4.2).

According to the participants, the clients' style of material interaction indicated the coping strategies they used most. Because art-making focuses on doing and experiencing rather than thinking, the material interaction style provided information about the clients' flexibility to explore and change their emotional and behavioral strategies.

In terms of the art product, art therapists were able to infer clients' material interaction based on the analysis of formal elements of clients' art products (see §2.6). Based on these formal elements, art therapists could describe clients' mental health in terms of their ability to attune and adapt to the properties of the art materials and their rational and emotional coping strategies.

These findings guided the research project toward the third study using constructivist grounded theory methodology. I wanted to gain a clearer understanding of art therapists' interpretation of the formal elements of art products created during art therapy evaluation. The literature on assessing formal elements in art therapy observation appeared to be inconsistent in terms of which formal elements to observe, how to operationalize them, and how to interpret them in terms of mental health. I wanted to know how art therapists described the mental health of adults and to identify exactly which formal elements of the art product art therapists observed in order to gain insight into the mental health of clients in clinical art therapy practice.

In terms of formal elements of the art product, art therapists primarily observed the presence or absence of the formal elements of movement, dynamic, contour, and repetition, the primary formal elements, in combination with color mixture, figuration, and color saturation, the secondary formal elements. The combination of the presence or absence of these formal elements constructed the structure and variation of the art product. Structure refers to the way in which the art product is organized, varying from clearly high to low structure. The presence of contour in combination with the absence of movement and dynamic led to art products with high structure, meaning that they were very organized. The structure of these art products could be enhanced by the presence of color saturation and the absence of color mixture.

The presence of movement and dynamic in combination with the absence of contour and repetition led to art products with low structure: they appeared to be chaotic. The structure of these art products could be weakened by the presence of color mixture and the absence of figuration.

Variation referred to diversity in one or more formal elements within the art product, such as diversity in contour existed when some aspects of the art product were clearly outlined and others were diffuse. Art products exhibited less variation when they were on the polarities of structure. Hence, art products that were extremely organized or chaotic showed less variation.

In terms of mental health, art therapists were reluctant to describe mental health in terms of psychopathology. They were more explicit about the client's capacities and strengths than about the client's mental problems. Two main concepts emerged: balance and adaptability. Balance (see §1.4.1) existed when feeling – allowing, experiencing, and expressing emotions – and thinking – cognitive control – were in proportion. In other words, clients who were able to experience, allow, and express their emotions in a way that did not overwhelm them were considered balanced. Clients who were unable to experience, tolerate, express, or regulate their emotions were rated as more imbalanced. This could occur if these clients had a very high tendency for cognitive control or, in contrast, were easily overwhelmed by their emotions due to difficulties in regulating emotions. Thus, balance could indicate "illness." Adaptability (see §1.4.2) referred to the client's strength and potential ability to achieve balance. It consisted of self-management, openness, flexibility, and creativity.

Regarding the formal elements of the art product, art therapists considered the formal elements of the art product to be an expression of the client's mental state. The combination of formal elements determined the structure and variation of the art product (see §2.6.2 and 2.6.3). They assumed that art products with a clear high or low structure indicated that the client was more imbalanced. Very highly structured art products were associated with an imbalance toward thinking. Very low-structured art products were associated with an imbalance toward feeling. Art products with variation indicated adaptability, as variation was associated with experimentation, exploration, playfulness, risk-taking, and discovery.

By observing the formal elements that determined the structure and variation of the art product, art therapists in this study were able to formulate an art therapy assessment in terms of balance and adaptability and formulate the focus of treatment. The treatment focus guided the choice of art interventions. In general, art therapists believed that clients with high cognitive control might benefit from more affective interventions, whereas clients with difficulty regulating their emotions might benefit from more cognitive interventions.

These findings raised the question of whether it would be possible to describe the formal elements in such a way that they could be rated objectively. In the art therapy literature, several previous attempts to measure formal elements of art products could be identified, resulting in a number of art therapy assessment instruments. However, these instruments have been seriously criticized regarding their reliability and validity. Therefore, I wanted to define clinically relevant formal elements that could be reliably described and analyzed and test their relationship to mental health. To do this, I conducted a fourth study using a mixed methods design. I went back to basics, to the art theories that originally developed the formal analysis of art products. These formal elements were defined on five-point Likert scales and tested for inter-rater reliability based on 137 art products from 80 clients. Inter-rater reliability ranged from moderate to substantial for all items except "texture," which had poor inter-rater reliability.

I compared these reliable formal elements with the formal elements that art therapists conceptualized as primary and secondary formal elements in clinical practice and found similarities in the primary formal elements movement, dynamic, and contour and secondary formal elements repetition, mixture of color, and color saturation.

According to the art therapists in Study 3, the combination of these formal elements mainly determined the structure and variation of the art product. Therefore, I tested their interrelatedness. These primary formal elements appeared to be interrelated in line with the combinations found in Study 3; the presence of contour in combination with the absence of movement and dynamic resulted in high structure and vice versa: the presence of movement and dynamic in combination with the absence of contour resulted in low structure.

In Study 3, art therapists found that very high and low-structured art products had less variation and that structure and variation indicated imbalance and adaptability. This would indicate that clients that made very high or low-structured art products were more imbalanced and less adaptive. We therefore tested whether the scores of the combination of these formal elements were related to scores on psychological complaints, resiliency, and experiential acceptance.

Findings showed that even though dynamic and movement significantly related to psychological complaints, the combination of movement, dynamic, and contour was not significant. The combination of the formal elements movement, dynamic, and contour significantly related to the scores on resiliency and experiential acceptance with the strongest relationship with experiential acceptance. Based on these results, the formal elements movement and dynamic indicated adult mental health more clearly in terms of what art therapists called "health" than in terms of what they called "illness." The combination of these formal elements accounts, statistically significantly, for 19% of the variance on the measure of resiliency and for 29% of experiential acceptance. This seems to be in line with the art therapists' perspective on mental health in which they emphasize the importance to assess the client's health in terms of adaptability, their flexibility, openness, self-management, and creativity. These findings therefore imply that the art form, specifically the combination of formal elements, is related to clients' coping strategies.

In relation to the ongoing discussion regarding the use of art form in art therapy assessment, three main findings emerged from this research project. First, the findings indicate that the art-making process and the art product appear to be related. Specifically, the client's material interaction during the art-making process is reflected in the formal elements of the art product. Second, a combination of a limited number of formal elements of the art product appears to be relevant as indicators of health. Finally, the findings suggest that the art form is more reflective of mental health than mental illness.

ArTA was developed based on the findings that the observation of material interaction, material experience, and the specific combination of formal elements of the art product make it possible to assess the client's balance between thinking and feeling and adaptability. These concepts, and how they relate to one another, are described further below.

2.2   A little history

In order to place the ArTA method in the international landscape and history of art therapy observation and assessment, it is important to take a look at this landscape.

The assumption that there is a relationship between mental health and the client's[2] art work[3] is the foundation of art therapy. The assumption is that the methodical use of art interventions contributes to mental health, and vice versa: (aspects of) mental health become visible in the art product(s). However, there are many different perspectives on what exactly this relationship looks like. These stem from different theoretical, historical, and practical approaches,[4] each with its own view of the role of the art process and the art product. Roughly speaking, a tripartite division can be made (see also Table 2.1).

In order to position the ArTA method in the international landscape and history of art therapeutic observation and assessment, it is important to examine it closely.

The first approach has its origins in psychodynamic or psychoanalytic theories. For decades, counselors have been fascinated by the drawings and paintings, or art products, of clients.

It has long been thought, especially by psychiatrists, that the art product, and especially its content, contains traces of the nature and severity of psychopathology. Within this approach, the art process is seen as a relationship of transference and countertransference between the client, the therapist, and the art product (e.g., Case & Dalley, 2014; Eisenbach et al., 2014; Gilroy & McNeilly, 2000; Schaverien, 1999, 2005).

According to this approach, art expression provides access to unconscious feelings, thoughts, and memories (Hilbuch et al., 2016). Transference takes place during the art process in the way that the client interacts with the material provided by the therapist and in the interaction between the client and the therapist. Not only is the therapist the object of transference, but the material is also considered an object of transference. Art materials play a central role because materials that are fluid, colorful, and bright invite the visualization of unconscious images, emotions, thoughts, and memories.

Table 2.1 Overview of different approaches in art therapy observation and assessment

Approach	Vision of the relationship art form and mental health	Examples of instruments/ methods for observation and assessment	Role of the art material	Scientific evidence
Art in therapy/ Analytical art therapy/ Art psychotherapy	Based on psychodynamic and analytic theories. The art-making process involves a transference and countertransference relationship between the client, the therapist, and the art product. The symbolic content of the art product is emphasized on the assumption that it reveals unconscious psychological conflicts of the client.	House Tree Person (HTP) Thematic Apperception Test (TAT)	The material is seen as an object of transmission. Materials that are fluid, colorful, and bright invite the visualization of unconscious images, emotions, thoughts, and memories. Testing is limited to drawing materials.	Little because of lack of reliability and validity due to subjectivity in interpreting the symbolic content of an art product.
Art-based therapy	Originally also based on psychodynamic theories, the focus shifts from symbolic content to formal elements related to psychopathology.	Diagnostic Drawing Series (DDS) Person Picking an Apple from a Tree (PPAT) and accompanying Formal Elements Art Therapy Scale (FEATS) Descriptive Assessment of Psychiatric Art (DAPA) Nürtinger Rating Scale (NRS)	Testing focuses on making one specific product with prescribed drawing materials.	Criticism of psychometric qualities of art-based instruments. These include diverse formal picture elements that are defined differently. Subjectivity also plays a role in interpreting scores. Vision of pathology is outdated.

(Continued)

Table 2.1 (Continued)

Approach	Vision of the relationship art form and mental health	Examples of instruments/ methods for observation and assessment	Role of the art material	Scientific evidence
Art as therapy/ Creative art therapy	Eclectic perspectives with emphasis on the therapeutic effect of the art form: the way a client reacts to different materials and assignments is seen as an expression of mental health (strengths). The art product, and especially the formal elements, is not directly related to symptoms of disorders but seen as the visual traces of the art-making process.	No specific methods or tests. Mainly how the client handles tasks, coping strategies used, frustration tolerance, and whether risk-taking is observed. Example is the Expressive Therapies Continuum (ETC).	Properties of art materials are theorized in which more solid materials are more likely to evoke a cognitive experience and fluid materials an affective one.	Little but promising research has been done.

In terms of the art product, this approach emphasizes the symbolic content. It assumes that it reveals unconscious psychological conflicts within the client (Hacking, 1999; Naumburg, 1966, 2001; Simon, 2001; Ulman & Bernard, 2001). According to this approach, the art product should also be seen as a transitional object through which the client, on an unconscious level, discusses experiences with himself and the therapist. Indeed, the content would express unexpressed feelings and thoughts about the therapist.

This is also the basic idea behind several projective drawing tests, such as the House-Tree-Person Test (HTTP) (Buck, 1948) and the Thematic Apperception Test (TAT) (Murray, 1943). These tests use only drawing materials. However, the scientific basis of this approach is very weak and has been seriously criticized. This is because of the lack of reliability and validity due to the subjectivity in interpreting the content of an art product (Betts, 2005, 2006, 2016; Betts & Groth-Marnat, 2014; Joiner et al., 1996; Schoch et al., 2017).

With the increasing emphasis on evidence-based practice, the focus has shifted from symbolic content to formal, more objective elements of art products such as line, color, and motion. This approach, also known as the art-based approach, assumes that the formal elements of the art product visually represent the client's art-making process. The evaluation of the formal elements is considered to be the most objective (Eytan & Elkis-Abuhoff, 2013; Gantt, 2001, 2004; Kaplan in Malchiodi, 2012; Kim et al., 2012; Mattson, 2009; Thomas & Cody in Gilroy et al., 2012; Thyme et al., 2013). The formal elements are said to represent the client's symptoms in accordance with disorders classified in the DSM or ICD (Cohen et al., 1986; Conrad et al., 2011; Elbing & Hacking, 2001; Gantt & Tabone, 1998; Hacking, 1999; Schoch et al., 2017; Stuhler-Bauer & Elbing, 2003).

Based on this approach, several diagnostic art-based instruments have been developed. These assess formal elements and relate them to symptoms of disorders. Examples include the Diagnostic Drawing Series (DDS) (Cohen et al., 1986, 1994), the Person Picking an Apple from a Tree (PPAT) (Gantt & Tabone, 1998), and the accompanying Formal Elements Art Therapy Scale (FEATS) (Gantt, 2001), the Diagnostic Assessment of Psychiatric Art (DAPA) (Hacking, 1999), and Nürtinger Rating Scale (NRS) (Elbing & Hacking, 2001). These tests focus on the production of a specific product using prescribed materials. For example, drawing a person picking an apple from a tree with a particular type of chalk. Although there is some research showing that scoring formal elements is promising in assessing clients' clinical state, there is also criticism of the scoring methods used (Betts, 2006; Nan & Hinz, 2012). This criticism is that these studies have mostly used inappropriate statistical methods to assess inter-rater reliability, which results in low reliability and validity of these instruments. In addition, each instrument assesses different formal elements, and when they assess the same formal image elements, they are defined differently. There is also increasing criticism of the focus on symptoms of disorders as classified in the DSM (see also §1.4).

The third approach, in contrast to the previous two, places more emphasis on the therapeutic effect of the art-making process itself. This approach is also referred to as art as therapy or creative art therapy (Betensky, 1973; Kramer, 1975; Lowenfeld, 1952; Naumburg, 1966; Rhyne, 1973; Rubin, 2009; Wadeson, 1980, 2002). This approach is more eclectic in nature and emphasizes the importance of both the art-making process and the art product. According to this approach, both are important in treatment as well as in art therapy observation and assessment. In particular, the way that a client responds to different art materials and tasks is seen as an expression of mental health. Thoughts, feelings, and behaviors are expressed that are less easily expressed in other, more verbal ways (Conrad et al., 2011; Hinz, 2009, 2015, 2020). The art product, and especially the formal elements, is not directly related to symptoms of disorders but seen as the visual traces of the art-making process (Hinz, 2009, 2015, 2020; Kagin & Lusebrink, 1978; Lusebrink, 2010).

On this basis, consideration is given as to whether the client could benefit from art therapy. In terms of the art product, this approach also emphasizes the formal elements. However, unlike the art-based approach, these are not directly related to symptoms of disorders (Chilton, 2013; Czamanski-Cohen & Weihs, 2016; Gussak & Rosal, 2016; Haeyen, 2018; Rankanen, 2016; Springham et al., 2012). Here, the formal elements are related to more general aspects of the client's health. Various humanistic, neuroscientific, developmental, and Gestalt theories are integrated. An example is the development of the Expressive Therapies Continuum (ETC) (Kagin & Lusebrink, 1978; Hinz, 2020). Research on this approach is still in its infancy, yet promising.

In short, there are different approaches with different arguments and emphases. Some approaches are not supported by science, and as a result, the methods of observation and assessment derived from them turn out to be unreliable and/ or invalid. The question then arises as to whether we want or even need to use them in practice with our clients.

It therefore seems difficult to develop reliable and valid methods for observation and assessment in art therapy. One factor that may play a role in this is the complexity of studying the art form and the relationship between the art form and mental health. Both concepts are complex in themselves and steeped in subjectivity, and even more so in relation to each other. This makes them difficult to explore. As an art therapist and health scientist, I have had the opportunity to peel back the layers of complexity and subjectivity. Through years of research, I have come to understand the relationship between the art form and mental health of adult clients. This has led to the development of the ArTA method.

2.3   ArTA

ArTA can be broadly positioned within the art as therapy approach described in the previous section. In fact, ArTA is based on the therapeutic effect of the art form, in which both the art-making process and the art product are important. Another similarity is that ArTA assumes that the way a client interacts with the art material is important. The (symbolic) content of the art product is not as significant, but *how* it is made, and this cannot be related to symptoms of classified disorders. What ArTA adds to this approach is an evidence-based specification of these assumptions. This shows that the art-making process does matter, specifically material interaction and material experience. We also know that the art product matters, specifically the combination of a specific set of limited formal elements that determine structure and variation. It also seems that material interaction, material experience, and art product are related and that these are related to mental health, specifically to balance between thinking and feeling, and to adaptability. The following sections describe the above in more detail.

2.4   Material interaction

Material interaction is how a person interacts with the properties of the art material during an art-making process. Material interaction is perhaps the most fundamental aspect of art therapy and ArTA. Consider that if a client does not interact with the art material, very little happens. In Chapter 1, we talked about structuring the art-making process through materials, techniques and tools, and instruction. When observing material interaction, it is especially important to look at how someone interacts with the material. It is about observable behavior when interacting with the art material. We observe different categories of material interaction, see Table 2.2.

When observing material interaction, it is important to consider the context of the art-making. Section 1.3 described how the different properties of materials, the technique and tools used, and the instruction determine the structure of an art-making process. For example, pencils tend to invite a lot of line work and less color mixing than, say, watercolors. If someone wants to make precise, straight, dense lines with watercolors, that shows different information than if someone does it with pencils. The instructions can also influence the art-making. For example, did the client choose the material or was it prescribed by the therapist? Were the possibilities of the material explained/demonstrated or not? Was a particular technique offered by the therapist or not? Therefore, it is important that the art therapist is aware of the components that influence the structure of art-making and thus determine the context of the session (see §1.3). Only then can the observed material interaction be interpreted correctly. For this reason,

Table 2.2 Categories of material interaction

Movement:	The size (small or large motions), the direction (outward or toward themselves), and the type of movement (curved, straight, vertical, or horizontal).
Pressure:	The amount of physical force that is applied (light or heavy) and the amount of focus (alert and attentive or nondirected).
Grip:	The way a client holds the art materials or tools. This can be loose or firm from the wrist or fingers.
Organization:	The way a client organizes the art-making (well-organized, systematic, or thoughtful versus chaotic or impulsive) and the activity (passive, coincidentally versus active or initiating).
Tempo:	The speed of art-making (slow versus fast).
Physical contact:	The contact that the fingers and hands make with the material during art-making (smearing, squeezing, rubbing, etc.) and the amount of contact (using the whole hand or more, using just the fingertips or no physical contact at all).
Rhythm:	The continuity of actions in time during the art-making (repetitious/continuous versus variable/interrupted).
Space:	The amount of space the art-making requires, related to the size of the canvas or paper and the amount of material that is used.
Lining:	Art-making can involve a large or a small amount of lining, and the type of lining (sketching versus outlining).
Mixing of color	The amount of mixing of colors during art making (a lot of mixing versus no mixing).
Shaping:	Removing or adding art materials in order to create shapes (adding or removing art material).
Dialogue:	The amount of exploration: exploring, making use of, experimenting, and playing with the properties of art materials.

the ArTA observation form (see Chapter 4 or Appendix 2) first notes the "context of the session."

It is also important to note that these categories alone have little or no diagnostic value. It is the combination of the different categories that indicates what characterizes a person's way of interacting with art material. We call this the material interaction style. After at least three sessions with different materials, a pattern can be observed. This gives a reliable assessment of what characterizes someone in material interaction. From the analogical thinking model (see §1.5), we know that the processes that drive material interaction are parallel to the processes that drive behavior in other situations. In other words, the way a person shapes and interacts with material says something, in a diagnostic sense, about the processes that drive behavior in situations outside of therapy. Both the style and pattern of material interaction are explained in the following subsections.

2.4.1 Style of material interaction

Material interaction style is the combination of the different categories of material interaction, such as movement, force, and speed (see Table 2.3). Together they give a picture of how a client interacts with the material. For example, exerting a lot of force combined with large movements, at a high tempo, with a loose wrist, lots of space, and little order gives a very different picture of a client's material interaction than exerting a lot of force combined with small movements, at a low tempo, with a firm grip, little space, and lots of order.

An example:

A client, an adult male, works with a B2 pencil on A4 paper (8 1/4 × 11 3/4 inches) on a landscape by example. He makes small, tight movements (*movement*), in an organized manner, first sketching the landscape in outline, then working out further details (*organization*). He works slowly (*tempo*), presses hard on the pencil (*pressure*), and holds the pencil with a steady wrist (*grip*). He takes up little space (*space*) and repeats (*rhythm*) the horizontal and vertical lines (*movement* and *lining*), which are often erased and reestablished (*shaping*) to make the landscape resemble the example as closely as possible (*organization*).[5] He makes little use of the characteristics of the B2 pencil, such as creating dark and light accents (*dialogue*).

Compare with this example:

A client, an adult male, works with charcoal with smooth, large circular movements without interruptions (*movement*). He works at a high speed (*tempo*) and exerts a lot of pressure on the material, sometimes breaking it (*pressure*). The lines (*lining*) repeat themselves (*rhythm*) and fill the entire 18 × 24 inches sheet of paper (*space*). He starts with an idea, which gradually gets lost as he becomes absorbed in the action (*organization*). He erases nothing, only adds lines

Table 2.3 Continuum of material interaction style

Rational Material Interaction	Affective Material Interaction
This style is characterized by thoughtfulness, precision, conscientiousness, control, and focus on the final result. Usually, a (thoughtful) plan is present.	This style is characterized by action orientation. Doing is central, where impulse or feeling are often the cause and/or predominate, and where there is usually no well-thought-out plan.

(*shaping*). He rubs the charcoal, first with the tip of his index finger, then with all fingers at once (*physical contact*). While this is appropriate to the properties of charcoal, he does not seem to be in contact with the material; the material seems to lead (*dialogue*) and he has no intention (*organization*) of exploring other possibilities (*dialogue*).

Each client will interact with the material in their own way during the art-making process, everyone has their own style of material interaction. However, we can place the style on a continuum from rational to affective (see Table 2.3).

Clients with a rational material interaction style tend to be planned, thoughtful, conscientious, precise, and in need of control. In addition to advantages in situations that require reflection, organization, and planning, an overly rational material interaction style can have disadvantages such as perfectionism and difficulty identifying, acknowledging, and expressing feelings.

An emotional material interaction style is characterized by, among other things, an action orientation. The doing itself is central, where the impulse or feeling is often the trigger and/or predominant, and where there is usually no thoughtful plan. Clients with an overly emotional material interaction style are easily overwhelmed by their feelings and may have difficulty regulating their feelings, structuring impulses, and dealing with boundaries.

Each client's material interaction style is unique, but it cannot be assessed based on a single session. This is because an event can be influenced by many factors unrelated to mental health per se, for example, familiarity with the material and an argument or difficult conversation prior to the art therapy session. Therefore, within ArTA, material interaction is observed on at least three occasions, preferably with different 2D materials. We then refer to this as a pattern of material interaction.

2.4.2 Patterns of material Interaction

The pattern of material interaction consists of the combinations of the material interaction categories that emerge over time. ArTA therefore does not rely on the observation of a single session: the client's material interaction is observed in at least three events, preferably when working with different 2D materials with different properties. Working with varied materials requires different actions based on material properties and techniques. A client may continue to apply or vary their material interaction style regardless of the material. Similarities in material interaction that transcend these differences are characteristic of the client's material interaction and therefore of diagnostic value. We call this the material interaction pattern.

An example:

Suppose the client from the first example in §2.4.1 works with pencil, chalk, and paint at three different times. In doing so, he repeatedly makes small movements, with a clear plan, at a slow pace, with a lot of lining. In this case, there is a rather rational pattern of material interaction because no matter what material this client is working with, he tries to maintain direction and control.

In practice, such a uniform pattern is not always present, and there is nuance and diversity. Typically, we can recognize three patterns. In the first pattern, the client tends to interact with the material more from cognition than from feeling. In the second pattern, the client tends to interact with the material more from impulse or feeling. And there is a third pattern, which we have not encountered much in the research on which ArTA is based, but which is mentioned here for completeness. In this pattern, the client alternates between interacting with the material more from cognition or more from affect. This does not mean that there are both rational and affective aspects to the material interaction, the material experience, and the structure and variation of the art product, but that there is an alternation between a clearly predominantly rational style of material interaction and a clearly predominantly affective style of material interaction.

There is another reason why the client is observed at least three times with different materials. This is because it allows assessment of how fixed a pattern is. If there is no variation in the way the client handles different materials at different times, then a pattern tends to be more fixed than if you observe some variation. For example, if the client in the first example in §2.4.1 still shows a rational material interaction even when working with colored ink and a wet-on-wet technique, then this pattern is more fixed than if this client can let go of some control and be tempted to let the material flow. The client in this case may want to maintain strong direction and control and is afraid, unwilling, or unable to look at what the material can do based on its properties. And in the case of the client in the second example, who tends toward an affective style of material interaction but still manages to structure when working with colored pencil, the pattern seems a little less fixed. This is also the power of observing material interaction; in addition to patterns of behavior that may have been the reason for asking for help, it also makes visible the (potential) developmental space and possibilities of the client. The less fixed the pattern, the more favorable the treatment prognosis.

A final important point when observing material interaction is that there are no measurable profiles, as each client is unique and has his or her own distinctive pattern of material interaction. This means that ArTA observes in an individual-centered way. For some clients, certain aspects of material interaction are more central than for others. The rational-affective continuum provides guidance in determining where the client is stuck and also where there is specific potential and room for development. This helps to formulate treatment goals that are realistic and tailored to the client, and to estimate the duration of treatment. In general, the less extreme and fixed a pattern of material interaction is, the more positive one can be about the duration, focus, and outcome of treatment. This is discussed further in Sections 2.8 and 2.12.

2.5   Material experience

Material experience is the way a client experiences the art material. Section 2.4 described how a client interacts with the properties of the art material in his or her own way, creating a personal experience. For example, a client may find the rubbing of a soft pastel very pleasant or, on the contrary, dirty and unpleasant. Positive and negative sensations and feelings can arise. The experience and perception of material interaction is often immediate without extended awareness. Observation of the material experience provides insight into how and to what extent the client can recognize, allow, appropriately express, and regulate feelings. This may include a distinction between positive and negative feelings.

Although each client's material experience is unique, we place it in the context of the session. In Section 1.3, it was described that the context of the session is determined by the structure of the art form. This is determined by the properties of the materials in combination with the technique, tools, and instruction. More solid materials and linear techniques tend to contribute more structure, especially if these materials are familiar. More fluid materials and pictorial techniques tend to produce less structure. The client's experience of the materials reflects the extent to which the client can let go of control or, on the contrary, finds it difficult to do so. Clients who find it difficult to let go and want to remain in control will experience a material that does not allow them to be controlled differently than clients who have less difficulty with this. In the first case, interacting with materials that are more difficult to control can cause tension or frustration. And in the second case, for example, playfulness and relaxation.

Observing material experiences also gives insight into how the client handles these. Are the feelings recognized? Are they allowed or avoided, or do they overwhelm the client? And how are the feelings expressed: verbally and/or non-verbally, for example through posture, facial expression, or otherwise? These observations should be placed in the context of the session (see §1.3). This makes it possible to see what factors might be influencing this; the characteristics of the material, the technique(s) and tools used, and the instruction. If so, it gives insight into any client preferences and the degree of structure in which feelings can be allowed and possibly further explored. This is also the reason why the context of the session is noted on the ArTA observation form (see Chapter 4 or Appendix 2). It is therefore important that the art therapist is well aware of the properties and possibilities of the art material. Only then can the observed material experiences be interpreted correctly.

An example:

Returning to the client from the first example in Section 2.4.1. Imagine the following:

As he draws a landscape with the B2 pencil, he is quietly present. He makes little contact with the therapist or other clients: all his attention is on the drawing. As time passes, he erases more and more lines, begins to sigh, and his posture becomes tense; his shoulders are hunched, and he hangs over his work on the edge of his chair. When the therapist asks how things are going, he indicates that he is unable to reproduce the example exactly. This annoys him. When the therapist mentions the frequent erasing, the client says that this is the worst of all: he cannot erase the lines. The therapist tells him to press the pencil less hard and to start a new sketch. This will make it easier to erase the lines and later determine which lines to press harder. The client tries this, and the tension eases. He can correct the lines more easily and look at his work with a little more distance and determine which lines he is happy with and which he is not. When the therapist asks how things are going, he sighs with relief and says, "Better!".

The difficulty in observing material experience is that it is not always externally visible. Of course, verbal expressions are important – what someone says, as well as sighing, falling silent, etc. – and nonverbal expressions, such as the client's facial expressions and posture during art-making, can be observed. The above example also shows that the therapist's observation makes it possible to name the observed behavior – in this case, erasing. In addition, it is important to actively check with the client what is being experienced, because not everything is outwardly visible. If this is not checked with the client, there is the potential to make wrong observations and interpretations. This can be done in the moment, as in the example, but also through reflection afterward (see §2.10).

Finally, the therapist's material knowledge and skills play an important role in observing the material experience. Many clients do not usually work in the visual arts or have not done so for a long time. As a result, many materials are unfamiliar. It is interesting to observe how clients deal with this. Do they choose familiar or unfamiliar materials? Do they try out the properties by doing, or do they like to get more explanation so that they have a sense of control? As an art therapist, it is important to be able to navigate this and, when necessary, provide the client with the right explanation of the material. Of course, this requires the therapist to know the materials inside-out.

Again, at least three observations, preferably with different materials, are necessary to recognize patterns.

2.6   Art product

The art product is the visible result of the art-making process. In ArTA, it is assumed that the formal elements of the art product reflect the material interaction. Research (see §2.1) shows that specific combinations of formal elements determine the structure and variation of the art product as a whole. The structure and variation are related to balance and adaptability as aspects of mental health (see §1.4.1 and §1.4.2). Before we discuss this in more detail, let us take a closer look at formal elements.

2.6.1 Formal elements

The analysis of formal elements has its origins in morphological art theory (Acton, 2009; De Visser, 2010; Van der Kamp et al., 2012). It emerged as a kind of counter-movement to iconological art analysis.

Iconological analysis of art is concerned with interpreting how the artist intended to convey a hidden or symbolic message through, for example, figuration, color, or composition. The artwork should be considered as a document that represents a certain zeitgeist (Panofsky, 1932, 1939). For example, the artwork represents the values and norms of a country, an era, a class, or a religious or philosophical perspective. This mode of analysis requires the viewer to have a certain amount of literary knowledge about the context in which the artwork was created, such as the spirit of the time, symbolism, and culture.

On the other hand, there is the morphological analysis of art. This focuses on the objective and visible formal elements such as line, color, shape, and movement that characterize the image (Acton, 2009; Boermans & van der Borght, 2017; Gale, 2016; Gerrits, 2018; Huntsman, 2016; Taylor, 2014; Wilson & Lack, 2016). Often these are positioned on a continuum of polarities, such as linear versus pictorial. This means that a formal element may be present to some degree. For example, an art product may contain a lot of, a little, or no line, movement, color, contour, etc.

The observation of formal elements is also used in art therapy. The underlying idea is that the formal elements reflect how the client has worked and wanted to express themselves. This would be related to mental health (e.g., Gilroy et al., 2012; Hinz, 2020). Based on this assumption, several art-based methods and measurement instruments for observation and assessment have been developed (see §2.2). However, these instruments have been criticized for limited reliability and validity (Betts, 2006; Claessens et al., 2016; Nan & Hinz, 2012; Schoch et al., 2017). This means that the way formal elements are defined in these measurement tools is not consistent and no clear relationship to mental health has been demonstrated. This is probably due to the lack of uniformity. Different formal elements are used, they are defined differently, and different views are held on how formal elements should be interpreted in terms of mental health. There is also criticism for the focus on psychopathology and there is a call for more emphasis on the client's strengths and abilities.

In the research on which ArTA is based I set out to find out what, if any, formal elements are actually related to mental health. First, I wanted to know which formal elements transcend different art theories. Next, I wanted to know how formal elements can be described in a way that they can be reliably observed. Finally, I tested which reliably-observable formal elements are related to mental health. It was important to know whether any formal elements are related to mental health at all and, if so, which ones and what exactly do they say about mental health? Are they related to symptoms and/or healthy aspects?

The focus here was on the formal elements of two-dimensional art products, because within art therapy and art therapy observation and assessment, drawing and painting materials are often used.

This revealed that the following formal elements are important to observe: movement, dynamic, contour, repetition, color mixing, and color saturation (see Table 2.4).[6] Based on the research, we can describe these in such a way that they can be analyzed reliably. This means that, based on these descriptions, two different people observing the same art product independently will come to the same conclusion.[7]

Table 2.4 outlines the formal elements. Appendix 1 contains the more detailed descriptions as used in the study.

As described at the beginning of this section, formal elements can be positioned on a continuum of polarities. For this reason, the formal elements in the ArTA study were elaborated on a 5-point scale. Here, 1 indicates no or minimal presence, and 5 indicates a high degree of presence of the formal element in question in the art product. This 5-point scale is intended to help analyze the formal elements of art products, and particularly if the analysis of formal elements is new, this can help to estimate the degree of presence of the formal elements. It is not a measurement tool.

Let's analyze an art product. Take a look at the right-hand image in Table 2.4 on repetition. This flower-like painting was made with watercolor at a size of 30 × 40 cm (12 × 15 inches). Little *movement* is present: we can recognize small movements that follow the direction of the shapes, without overlap. If we were to rate this using the 5-point scale as in the ArTA study (see Appendix 1), you would score a 2.

There is little *dynamic*[8] present: there is no tension at all in the art product. The art product shows calmness, a peaceful coexistence between the image itself and the space around it, all elements of the art product remain entirely within the frame. The dynamic is characterized by complete tranquility. If we were to rate this using the 5-point scale as in the ArTA study (see Appendix 1), you would score a 1.

The art product has a lot of *contour*: the shapes are sharply delineated, as if they have been "cut out." If we were to rate this using the 5-point scale as in the ArTA study (see Appendix 1), you would score a 5.

The art product has a lot of *repetition*: the art product contains distinct rhythmic patterns. All the colors and shapes recur four times in a predictable pattern. They characterize the art product as a whole. If we were to rate this using the 5-point scale as in the ArTA study (see Appendix 1), you would score a 5.

There is no *mixture of color* in the art product. Colors in the art product are separate from each other. If we were to rate this using the 5-point scale as in the ArTA study (see Appendix 1), you would score a 1.

There is a lot of *color saturation*. All the colors in the art product are almost fully saturated, but some of the paper is still visible. If we were to rate this using the 5-point scale as in the ArTA study (see Appendix 1), you would score a 4.

Table 2.4 Description and illustrations of the formal elements in ArTA

Movement	The amount and direction of movement in the art product, ranging from little to a large amount. Movement is evident in the brushstroke/linework.	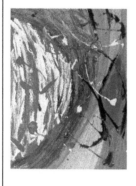 The art product has almost no movement. Small movements can be recognized in the brushstroke/linework, in mostly the same direction, without overlap.	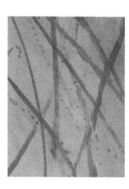 The art product has a lot of movement; many and/or large movements in different directions can be recognized in the brushstroke/linework, and there may be overlap.
Dynamic	The tension in the image, ranging from little to a large amount. It reflects the vitality of the movement.	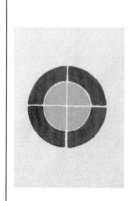 There is no tension at all in the art product. The image exhibits a peaceful coexistence with the space around it. All elements of the art product remain entirely within the frame.	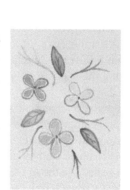 There is a great deal of tension between image and frame. The art product is completely and utterly frame-deprived; the image seems to be restrained with friction by the frame. The dynamic is restless and turbulent.

Contour

The degree of delineation of parts of the visual product by outlining or tightly placing shapes against each other, ranging from little to a large amount.

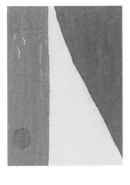

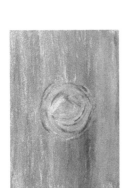

There is little contour. Some surfaces can be recognized, but the delineation is not sharp, rather sketchy, friable, or affected.

An image has a lot of contour when shapes are completely outlined and/or sharply delineated, as if they have been "cut out." The work then looks linear.

Repetition

The degree to which one or more elements are repeated in a pattern, ranging from few to many.

An image with little repetition has little rhythm and no clear pattern.

The art product contains one or more distinct repeated patterns. These patterns concern all elements of the art product. They characterize the art product as a whole.

(Continued)

Table 2.4 (Continued)

Mixture of color	The degree to which colors are visibly mixed, ranging from none to a large amount.	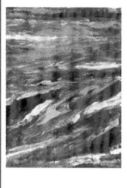 In an image with no color mixing, the colors are applied separately.	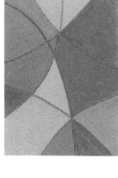 In an image with a lot of mixture of color, most of the colors are visibly mixed.
Color saturation	The degree of saturation, ranging from little to a large amount.	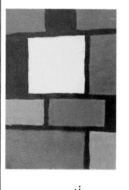 The image has little color saturation if the material is applied thinly or transparently, leaving much of the carrier still visible.	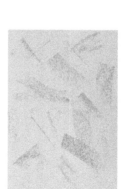 The image has a lot of color saturation when the material is thick, even impasto, and the carrier cannot be seen.

When analyzing formal elements of an art product, it is important to consider the context of art-making. Section 1.3 described how different properties of materials, the technique and tools used, and instruction determine the structure of the art-making process. These also influence the observation of formal elements.

For example, it is more obvious that contour is present in an art product if it has been drawn with a highlighter than if it has been done with a thick bamboo brush and watercolor. There will also be a difference in color mixing. It is important to take this into account when determining the extent to which a formal element is present. This requires a great deal of knowledge about the properties of art materials.

Instruction may also affect the extent to which a formal element is present. For example, were the possibilities of the material explained or not? Were techniques and/or tools prescribed or not? Therefore, when observing formal elements, it is important to consider the context of the art-making. For this reason, to illustrate the polarities of the formal elements in Table 2.5, two art products made with the same material were always used. This is also the reason why on the ArTA observation form (see Chapter 4 or Appendix 2) the material used is noted under "context of the session." Therefore, it is important that the art therapist is aware of the properties, possibilities and possible influences of art material, technique, tools, and instruction.

Furthermore, it seems that the individual formal elements influence each other: they can reinforce or weaken each other. For example, the contour in the art product is strengthened when there is little color mixing present and weakened when there is a lot of color mixing. The specific combination of formal elements determines the structure and variation of the art product as a whole.

2.6.2 Structure

The structure of an art product concerns the way the image is organized. It is determined by the combination of formal elements. We can place the degree of structure on a continuum from high structure to low structure. An art product with high structure looks more organized and contrived, whereas an art product with low structure looks more chaotic.

Considering Image 2.1, we see art products from two different adult female clients. Both art products are 30 × 40 cm (12 × 15 inches). They were made with acrylic paint, without instruction; the clients were allowed to decide what they wanted to create. Prior to making this art product, both clients had already attended two sessions of art therapy. The possibilities of the material had already been explained to them during these sessions.

What can you say about the formal elements of movement, dynamic, and contour in both products (see Table 2.4)? Based on this, what can you say about the degree of structure? And what can you say about the formal elements of repetition, mixture of color, and color saturation? Do they strengthen or weaken the structure? Try to answer these questions one at a time before reading on.

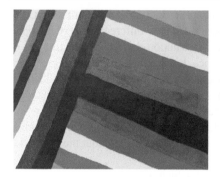 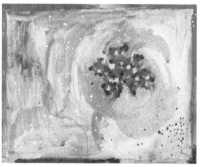

Image 2.1 Art products with high structure (left) and low (er) structure (right).

In the art product on the left, we see color planes/stripes that are applied evenly, tightly, parallel with small movements in only two directions. This creates little *movement* in the image. The planes of color are placed diagonally, and while this creates some tension in the image, the vitality of the movement remains rigid: the *dynamic* is static. The color planes are close together, so there is a lot of *contour* in the image. On this basis, the art product appears structured.

In addition, we see that the color planes are placed almost symmetrically to each other. This creates *repetition* in the image. The color is applied thickly. This results in high *color saturation*. There is no *mixture of color*. The presence of a lot of repetition and a lot of color saturation and the absence of mixture of color strengthen the structure of this art product. In conclusion, we can observe a lot of structure in this art product.

In the art product on the right, we see flowing organic lines and planes of varying size and direction. This creates *movement* in the image; the agile, almost tangled brushstroke is evident. The vitality of this movement is alive, creating *dynamic*. The whole image is framed by a colored stripe. The framing demarcates and thus creates a *contour*. On this basis, the art product appears less structured than the one on the left, but not completely unstructured. Slightly off-center in the ochre circle are dots of unmixed primary colors. This creates some *repetition* in the painting. We also see some repetition in the color gradient in the frame. The dots, splashes, and frames have been applied thickly, giving them a high *color saturation*. The other pastel parts were applied transparently and therefore have low *color saturation*. With the exception of the thick dots, the paint has been blended into the circular shape, creating a *mixture of colors*. In conclusion, this art product has less structure than the one on the left, but it is not completely unstructured.

As you can see in the examples above, the combination of formal elements determines the structure of the art product. We know from research (Pénzes, 2020; Pénzes et al., 2018) that this very structure is related to mental health. Although each art product is unique, specific combinations of formal elements

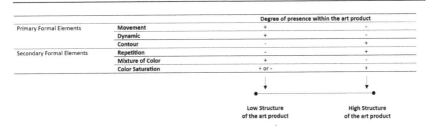

		Degree of presence within the art product	
Primary Formal Elements	Movement	+	-
	Dynamic	+	-
	Contour	-	+
Secondary Formal Elements	Repetition	-	+
	Mixture of Color	+	-
	Color Saturation	+ or -	+
		Low Structure of the art product	High Structure of the art product

Figure 2.1 How the combination of formal elements determines the degree of structure of the art product.

determine the degree of structure. Specifically, the combination of the formal elements movement, dynamic, and contour is the most important. We call these the primary formal elements. The combination of little movement, little dynamic, and a lot of contour indicates more structure in the art product. In contrast, the combination of high movement, high dynamic, and low contour indicates less structure (see Figure 2.1).

This impression of the structure of the art product is further strengthened or weakened by the formal elements of repetition, mixture of color, and color saturation which we call secondary formal elements. Thus, the structure of the art product can be strengthened by high repetition, low mixture of color, and high color saturation, and the structure is (further) weakened by low repetition and high mixture of color. Color saturation is a bit trickier at this point, as both high and low saturation can weaken the texture. High saturation can weaken the texture if, for example, there are thick, impasto blobs of paint. Low saturation can weaken the texture if, for example, there is a lot of transparency in the image due to the use of fluid materials or dry brush strokes. Again, the material used affects the interpretation of formal elements.

Thus, the structure of the art product depends on the combination of formal elements and can be placed on a continuum from low to high structure. The line under structure in Figure 2.1 illustrates this. Based on observation of one art product, a relationship with mental health has already been demonstrated. However, it is preferable to observe at least three art products, preferably made of different materials, to reveal patterns. The pattern of structure is related to the client's balance and adaptability (see §2.8).

In addition to being able to say something about the structure of the art product based on the formal elements, we can also say something about the variation of the art product.

2.6.3 Variation

Variation refers to the diversity in the formal elements of an art product. Like material interaction and art product structure, variation is observed at least three times. Observation across multiple art products provides insight into patterns of variation. These patterns can be placed on a continuum from many to few.

Look again at the two art products in Image 2.1 of §2.6.2. In the left art product, there is little variation: the movement, dynamic, contour, repetition, mixture of color, etc., are equally present or absent throughout the art product. In the art product on the right, more variation is seen: there are different movements, the dynamic is slightly more vivid even though the parts are not related, and there are different degrees of color saturation through both the use of dilution and impasto.

We saw in the previous section that the structure of an art product can be arranged on a continuum from low to high. Art products that are extremely structured or extremely unstructured tend to have less variation. Consider the two art products in Image 2.2. Both were created with colored ink by adult female clients. Both art products are 30 × 40 cm (12 × 15 inches). Both were made without instruction, where the clients were allowed to use all the materials available in the art therapy room.

In the art product on the left, pink- and blue-colored ink was applied with lots of water. Horizontal lines, splashes, and drops have created *movement* in the image. These go beyond the frame and add to the *dynamic* of the image. There are few clearly delineated shapes to be recognized, the image is pictorial and has little *contour*. Based on this combination of the formal elements of movement, dynamic, and contour, we observe low structure in the image. This is further weakened by the relatively high level of *mixture of color* and *color saturation*,[9] and the lack of a clear focus in the composition, resulting in little *repetition* in the image.

In the art product on the right, we see little *movement*. The *dynamic* is calm, there is no tension in the image. The shapes do not touch anywhere, the colors are separate: there is no *mixture of colors*. The leaves are outlined, and the flowers have a clear line. This creates *contour*. The very low degree of movement and dynamics combined with the high degree of contour contribute to a lot of structure in this art product. This is enhanced by the fact that the colored ink was applied without the addition of water, so there is a lot of *color saturation* and

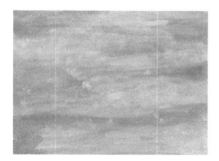 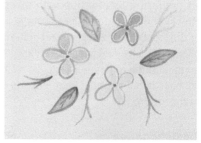

Image 2.2 Art products with low structure (left) and high structure (right) contain less variation.

little *mixture of color* in the image. There is also a certain amount of *repetition* in the shapes, which makes the composition nonrhythmic, but with a clear focus.

The left art product could be positioned on the structure continuum toward the low polarity. The right art product on the polarity high. There is little variation in both art products. In the left image, the colored ink is set with water. Here, we see horizontal movement where paint and water have been applied in layers. There are splashes here and there. This characterizes the entire art product and creates little variation in the formal elements of movement, dynamic, contour, repetition, color saturation, and mixture of color. These are consistent throughout the art product.

In the image on the right, we can see that the colored ink has not been applied mixed or diluted with water. As a result, the color saturation is the same throughout. Because the colors are not mixed anywhere, there is no variation in the color mix; all the shapes are outlined, so the outline is the same everywhere. It can be concluded that if a client shows a pattern with extremely high or extremely low structure in the art product, there will be less variation.

Compare the two art products in Image 2.3. Both art products were created by two different adult male clients who were instructed to paint a landscape with acrylic paint on paper. The size of the imagery is 40 × 50 cm (15 × 20 inches).

You can now see from the combination of formal elements that both art products contain some degree of structure: in both there is movement and dynamic combined with relatively little contour. There is a degree of repetition in both art products without being completely symmetrical. There is mixture of color and color saturation in both art products.

Looking more closely at these formal elements, we see that there is more variation in both art products than in the two art products in Image 2.2. There are different movements: small, large, short, long, horizontal, diagonal, straight, and curved. There are differences in mixture of color (more in the right art product than in the left): the colors were applied separately and mixed on paper. And

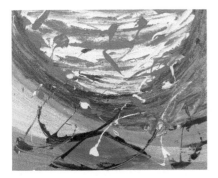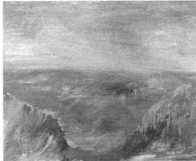

Image 2.3 Art products with less extreme low or high structure contain more variation.

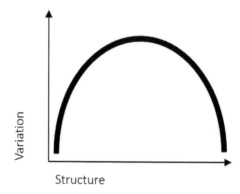

Figure 2.2 Extreme low and extreme high structure of an art product is related to less variation.

there are differences in color saturation: some parts are fully saturated, others are transparent.

In short, the less extreme the structure, the more variation. Figure 2.2 shows this schematically. You can see that the polarities of the structure are associated with little variation, and that as the structure moves away from the polarities, more variation appears. You can see a kind of "optimum." Theoretically, this could be said to indicate health. More on this in §2.8.

2.7   Relationship between material interaction, material experience, and art product

Material interaction, material experience, and art product are related. Material interaction is largely visible in the combination of formal elements that determine the structure and variation of the art product.[10]

This is represented by the right arrow in Figure 2.3. Material interaction also leads to material experience. This is the left arrow in Figure 2.3. We zoom in on this relationship a little further.

An example:

Two adult clients both work with acrylic paint. In Image 2.4, you can see each client's art product. Both art products measure 40 × 50 cm (15 × 20 inches). What can you say about the formal elements (see Table 2.4)?

There is little movement in the left art product. In the brush stroke, we see short, mostly horizontal movement. There is also some repetition, but the image is not symmetrical. The dynamic is quiet, almost static. There is a lot of contour in the art product, as the shapes are close together. We also see a high degree of color saturation: the paint has been applied thickly. There is no mixture of colors: the colors are applied directly from the pot, separately from each other.

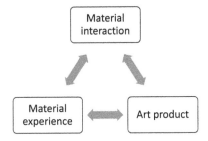

Figure 2.3 Relationship between material interaction, material experience, and art product.

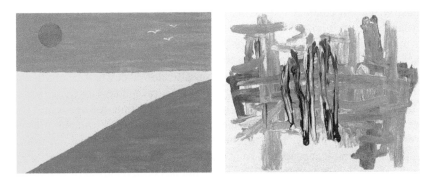

Image 2.4 Different categories of material interaction become visible in formal elements.

This combination of formal elements gives a structured impression of the art product as a whole (see §2.6.2).

The art product on the right shows a fair amount of movement, especially in the horizontal and vertical directions. The dynamic is energetic and powerful, and although the color does not go beyond the frame, there is some tension in the image. There is some contour, especially in the foreground and background, but it is significantly less than in the art product on the left. Color saturation is high: the paint has been applied in thick layers, and as these are scratched and wiped away here and there, impasto is created. There is a lot of mixture of color. The combination of these formal elements makes this art product seem more impulsive, but not completely chaotically structured (see §2.6.2).

What can you say about the structure of the art product based on these formal elements? And what about the material interaction of these clients (see Table 2.2)?

The art product on the left has relatively high structure due to the combination of low movement and dynamic, high contour, some repetition, low mixture of color, and high color saturation. In terms of material interaction, the client made relatively small movements, applied little pressure, and probably worked from a fixed grip and at a not too fast tempo. There appears to have been no physical contact with the material; no traces of fingerprints or smudges are visible. The action was probably repetitive, with mostly horizontal movements. Little line and color blending was used. It is difficult to say anything about the forms category. Assuming the material, and knowing that there was no pencil or eraser, it seems to have been mainly added. There is little dialog: the material is used in the same way throughout, and the maker seems to want to control the material by working with it precisely. In terms of structure, the work seems to have been done in a thoughtful, precise, and focused manner. On this basis, we could speak of a more rational style of material interaction.

The art product on the right is slightly less structured. It is a little more impulsive, but not completely chaotic. This is based on a lot of movement and dynamic (which is limited), little but some contour, quite a lot of repetition, a lot of mixture of color, and a lot of color saturation. In terms of material interaction, the client made larger movements in the art product on the right. A lot of pressure was used at a faster pace, but the action was also slowed down. A firm grip was probably used. There did not appear to be any physical contact with the material. The action was probably repetitive, based on the repetition of horizontal and vertical lines. Space was taken up, the entire paper was used, and the material was applied very thickly. The movement created a mixture of lines and colors. In terms of form, it appears that paint was mostly added although in some parts of the art product it can also be seen that paint has been removed by scratching or scraping. Little dialogue is visible. The material has been used in the same way throughout. In terms of structure, the work seems to have been done less thoughtfully and impulsively, with little focus, but with a conscious "stop" to the action. On this basis, we can speak of a more affective style of material interaction. The action, the doing, seems to have been central.

The above examples show that a high structured art product usually correlates with a more rational material interaction, and vice versa: low structure in the art product correlates with a more affective material interaction. In practice, however, it is never this black and white. An art product is never fully structured or unstructured and the material interaction is never completely rational or affective. It is important to place structure and material interaction on a continuum, based on the combination of formal elements and aspects of material interaction. In the case of structure, from high to low, and in the case of material interaction, from rational to affective. This also means that while an art product with a lot of structure indicates a more rational style of material interaction, it may still contain affective elements. The less extreme the structure and material interaction style, the more of these aspects you will be able to observe.

In addition, Section 2.6.3 described how the degree of structure is related to the degree of variation. Extremely structured and extremely unstructured art products tend to have less variation. The degree of variation is related to the core dialogue aspect of material interaction.

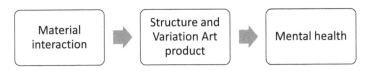

Figure 2.4 Relationship between material interaction, structure, and variation of the art product and aspects of mental health.

Look again at the two art products in Image 2.3. You can see from the variation present that there was more dialogue in the material interaction than in the art products in Image 2.2. There was painting, wiping, splashing (left), stamping (right). Variation is therefore associated with experimentation, exploration, playfulness, risk-taking, and discovery. Variation is therefore related to the client's level of imbalance and ability to adapt. In short, structure and variation of the art product are related to material interaction (see Figure 2.4). These, in turn, are related to specific aspects of mental health. Section 2.7 discusses this further.

In addition to the connection between material interaction and the art product, there is also a connection between material interaction and material experience. The properties of the art material being worked with and the way the client interacts with it create an experience.

Section 1.3 described how materials can be placed on a continuum from solid to fluid based on their properties, and that solid materials contribute to more structure in art design and fluid materials contribute to less structure.

Clients with a rational style of material interaction tend to want to control materials. They are generally more likely to choose solid materials because they are easy to control. Interacting with more fluid materials, which allow for less grip and control, will result in a different material experience. In addition, clients with a rational style of material interaction often have difficulty recognizing, acknowledging, and/or expressing feelings.

Clients with an affective style of material interaction, on the other hand, tend to have a little more difficulty in exercising control and are more likely to be guided or even overwhelmed by fluid materials that are less easily controllable. Clients with an affective style of material interaction will typically have a little more difficulty regulating their emotions. In short, material interaction leads to material experience and provides insight into any imbalance in thinking and feeling.

2.8 The relationship between material interaction, material experience, art product, and mental health

As described in Section 2.7, there is a correlation between material interaction, material experience, and the structure and variation of the art product. When a pattern of high structure is observed in a client's art products, there is usually a rational pattern of material interaction. Clients with rational material interaction like to be in control – in situations outside of therapy, but also when interacting with the art material. Depending on the context of the session in which this is more or less successful, this will determine the material experience in which sensing, recognizing, acknowledging, and expressing feelings can be difficult. With these clients there is usually an imbalance toward thinking.

If there is a pattern of low structure in the art product, there is usually an affective pattern of material interaction. Clients with affective material interaction, on the other hand, tend to have difficulty controlling their feelings. They are more likely to be guided or even overwhelmed by feelings – in situations outside of therapy, but also in interaction with art material. Depending on the context in which this is more or less the case, this will determine the material experience in which adequate expression and regulation of feelings through cognitive control may be difficult. In these clients, there is usually an imbalance toward feeling.

When the pattern of structure of the art product is positioned more on the polarities of the continuum (extremely high structure or extremely low structure), the pattern of material interaction will be more fixed and the material interaction will be more clearly rational or affective. As a result, there will be more imbalance – with a rational material interaction style toward thinking and with an affective material interaction towards feeling. We have already seen in Chapter 1 that both thinking and feeling are important for mental health. We also saw that processes in art-making are analogous to those that influence behavior in everyday situations.

Clients with a rational material interaction and an imbalance in thinking will therefore want to maintain control and direction in other situations. This also affects how they deal with uncontrollable situations.

Clients with an affective material interaction and an imbalance toward feeling will also have difficulty regulating impulses and feelings in situations outside of therapy. This also affects how they deal with a variety of situations and life events. This can lead to distress and cause them to seek help.

In practice, clients often emphasize these complaints. However, aspects of (potential) health, namely adaptability, can also be observed in the material interaction, material experience, structure, and variation of the art product. In fact, it is rare that patterns of structure are so extreme and unambiguous.

For example, the structure of an art product may be predominantly high – indicating a rational material interaction – and yet show some movement or vitality in its dynamic. In this case, there is also some variation. And it is this variation in the art product that indicates that the degree of imbalance is not extreme and that there is to some degree adaptability.

Understanding this helps not only in formulating an art therapeutic assessment, but also in determining whether and which art interventions are most appropriate to restore balance (see §2.12).

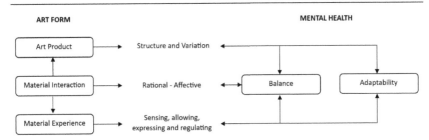

Figure 2.5 Relationship between material interaction, art product, and material experience with balance and adaptability.

Material interaction, material experience, and the structure and variation of the art product are thus interrelated and provide insight into any imbalance between thinking and feeling (in what direction and to what extent) and (potential) adaptability. The more fixed these patterns are, the greater the imbalance and the lower the adaptability. The opposite is also true: the less fixed these patterns, the less imbalance and the more adaptability. The above is summarized in Figure 2.5.

2.9   Role of instruction

Chapter 1 described how the context of art-making is determined by the properties of the materials, the techniques and tools used, and the instruction (see §1.3). The sections on material interaction (§2.4), material experience (§2.5), and the formal elements of the art product (§2.6) described their influence on observation of these aspects. With regard to the role of instruction, it was mentioned that it makes a difference whether a material is chosen by the client or provided by the art therapist; whether the possibilities of the material were explained or not; and whether the technique was instructed or determined by the client. This section elaborates on the role of instruction in ArTA.

Unlike most other observation methods (see Table 2.1), ArTA does not work with a standard prescribed assignment accompanied by a specific material. In this respect, ArTA can be integrated into the observation and assessment that takes place in regular practice. Even if the art therapist is part of a treatment team using a particular method or therapeutic approach, ArTA can be applied. Some art therapists see clients individually or in groups, and ArTA can still be used in these situations.

However, it is preferable that the client be affectively or cognitively guided as little as possible. Awareness of the influence of instruction and the use of materials and techniques is therefore important, in order to interpret the observation of the material interaction, the material experience, and the art product. Ideally, the client should be encouraged to start an art-making process with as few instructions as possible. This allows the observation to be as open as possible and provides insight into the client's material preferences, the client's need for structure, the client's patterns of material interaction across different materials, and how these are experienced. It is by no means the intention to throw the client in at the deep end. The role of the therapist is to connect very well with the client at the beginning of the observation and assessment and to evaluate what guidance is needed to create the necessary safety. This requires an open approach that balances the relationship between providing safety and providing space to see the client's most authentic behavior. This relationship shifts to three sessions of observation, the minimum number of sessions observed to determine the client's balance and adaptability.

For a client beginning art therapy, many materials will be unfamiliar. Some materials may be reminiscent of school days and may be associated with positive or negative feelings and expectations. In ArTA, the first observation session begins with an overview of all the materials available. It is not necessary to have a lot of different materials; however, it is important to have materials that cover the continuum from solid to fluid (see Figure 1.3). For example, it is important to have pencil, chalk, paint, and colored ink for the client to choose from. The materials are briefly described, and the properties of the materials are briefly mentioned, as well as the technical possibilities and the tools needed. The classification into solid/linear/graphic materials and fluid/pictorial/painting materials provides guidance, also to avoid overwhelming the client with information and unnecessary details. This explanation can be supported by examples, such as art products that may already be hanging in the therapy room, a demonstration of the material and technique, an overview file of materials and techniques, or otherwise.

Clients also regularly ask what the therapist can see in the art product; there is sometimes a sense of mystery about it. It can be important, therefore, to discuss clearly with the client the purpose of this phase of the treatment, which is to gain insight together into what is happening, and whether and how the treatment can be moved forward. By involving the client and showing that the client is seen as an individual, much of the mystery is removed. It is up to the therapist to decide how much of the ArTA method is explained in the process. In principle, this is not necessary and can vary from client to client. The therapist's own expertise determines this judgment.

Preferably, in the first observation session, the client is asked to choose from a wide arsenal of two-dimensional (2D) materials and work with them in their own way. The goal is to observe the client's preferences and how the client structures his or her art-making. This says a lot about how the client prefers to deal with other (everyday) situations. Some are more structured, thoughtful, organized, and make a plan that is executed step by step, while others are less structured, impulsive, chaotic and start without a (fully thought-out) plan and see how things go. It is also important to observe the degree of control a client needs to start an art-making process. Some clients need more guidance from the therapist than others.

For this first session, the client is asked to choose a material that appeals to them. This can be a material that is familiar to them, or a material that piques their curiosity. The client is informed that they can decide what to do with the material. A client may find it difficult to decide what to make, for example, because for various reasons we don't yet know at this point, no ideas come to mind, or just too many. In this case, the therapist can help by offering more structure (see also §1.3) by providing a theme, an example or even a sketch/coloring picture, etc. The different levels of art-making can be helpful here: copying (such as tracing over an example), imitating (such as using another picture as inspiration/ help), and experimenting (determining the form yourself and trying out the possibilities of the material).

The goal of this first step in ArTA is to gain insight into the client's preferences and the degree of structure the client needs to start an art-making process. In short, start as open and attuned to the client as possible to observe as many authentic client choices and behaviors as possible. It requires a balance between providing the minimum amount of structure for the client in question and at the same time providing enough structure to create a safe space within which the client can interact and experience. This also means giving few but sufficient instructions during the art-making to keep the situation safe. This is further explored in Chapter 3. On this basis, the material interaction, the material experience, and the art product can then be observed. In this initial session of observation, a first impression is created.

If clinical practice does not allow one to begin with such open observation, then this is not a problem. This could be the case, for example, when individual sessions alternate with group work in art therapy. It is then important to take into account the structure provided by the therapist when observing and interpreting.

In the second observation session, the instruction of the first observation session is repeated, except that the client is explicitly asked to choose a different material. By having the client work with a different material, it is possible to observe which aspects of material interaction, material experience, and art product recur and which do not.

It can be difficult when the art product started in the first observation session is not yet finished, especially if the client really wants to finish. It is preferable to start a new art product in the second observation session with a different material. If this is really problematic, which is also an interesting observation, it can be decided to give the client the opportunity to finish this art product first. The second observation session is the session in which the client starts a new process and product. It takes the expertise of the art therapist to make this judgment. This means that the first sessions of observation may consist of several sessions. However, it is advisable to ensure that a second and third observation session can take place within the time available for observation and assessment (often determined by the institution/department/therapy program).

Another point to consider is if the client chooses a material in the second observation session that is very similar in characteristics to the material chosen in the first observation session. For example, if the client chose pencil in the first observation session and colored pencil in the second. Or gouache and acrylic. If the client has a strong preference for the same material, a different technique with this material may be used. For example, if the client worked with soft pastel in the first session and wants to work with pastel chalk in the second session. If the colors were not blended in the first session, you may want to ask the client to rub out the chalk in the second session and to make the transitions between the colors. You can vary the instruction that determines the degree of structure. For example, you can leave it very open or direct it a bit more.

Observing the client's choice of materials gives a first impression of the client's preferences. For example, does the client choose materials that are familiar, materials that are easy to control and direct, or does the client choose materials that are new and arouse curiosity? Will the client choose similar materials in the second session or will the client look for a material with different characteristics? How much guidance does the client need from the therapist?

Also, observing material interaction, material experience, and the art product when working with different materials also provides a first impression of patterns. For example, regardless of the material, is the client more likely to engage in rational material interaction? Does a more fluid material make it easier for the client to sense bodily signals and feelings, or does it remain difficult? These first impressions guide the instruction in the third observation session.

In the third observation session, the client is stimulated and invited to interact in a different way than in the first two sessions. To do this, the therapist adjusts the instructions. Rather than leaving the instruction as open-ended as possible, the therapist provides those materials, techniques, and tools that enable the client to achieve different material interaction, material experience, and art product.

For example, a client who in the first two sessions seemed to have a more rational material interaction style with a preference for solid materials may now be given a choice of materials that are somewhat more fluid and less easily controlled. Or a client who made small movements on a relatively small-sized surface is invited to work on a larger-sized paper.

There is no intention at this stage to confront the client or take them completely out of their comfort zone. Therefore, materials with properties that are completely at the other end of the continuum are not offered. However, the goal is to encourage the client to try something different in a safe context. This can be done through a technical explanation of the material, technique, or tool. The goal is to gain insight into how fixed patterns are and what the client might need to restore balance and enhance adaptability. Table 2.5 briefly summarizes the instructions and associated goals.

Table 2.5 Instructions in ArTA

	Instructions	Goals
First Observation	Giving an overview of available 2D materials. The classification of solid/linear materials and fluid/pictorial materials provides guidance. Explanations may be supported with examples (see text). Explain the purpose and method of this phase of treatment. Ask the client to make a choice of materials and work with them in their own way. During art-making, provide minimal but sufficient instruction to keep the situation safe. Provide minimal but necessary structure (imitate, copy, experiment).	Providing client safety, familiarizing them with space, materials, and opportunities. Attuning expectations to the client. Observing material preferences, the way in which the client structures the art-making and the degree of guidance needed. Observing material interaction style, material experience, and structure and variation of the art product.
Second Observation	Same instruction as the first observation session, with the difference that the client is explicitly asked to choose a different material or technique.	Observe recurring aspects of material interaction style, material experience, and structure and variation of the art product.
Third Observation	Limit material selection based on observations from the first and second observation sessions.	Encouraging the client, within a safe context, to try something different to gain insight into how fixed patterns are. What keeps recurring regardless of the material used? These are patterns in material interaction, material experience, and structure and variation of the art product.

2.10 Role of reflection

The role of reflection was not explicitly explored in the research on which ArTA is based. Nevertheless, reflection with a client can be valuable soon after each session, but also after the observation and assessment over a minimum of three sessions has been completed. Reflecting on the process with the client provides more insight into the client's capability to reflect as into the client's perspective. This is in line with the individual-centered nature of ArTA. Observations made during the art process can also be evaluated with the client. Specifically, the experience of materials is an aspect that can be discussed, as this is not always fully visible during the creation of the art product (see §2.5).

Brief moments of reflection allow the client to step back from the art-making process. By reflecting together on the art product, the material interaction, and the material experience, the client can become aware of possible patterns and whether these are recognizable for functioning outside of therapy. What does the client encounter in everyday situations such as work and family? What might be different and why?

By listening to the client's experiences, preferences, wishes, ideas, expectations, and needs, the client is involved in the observation and assessment; what is going on, what is in the foreground, what is urgent, etc. This makes the client an active partner, including in any follow-up treatment. This benefits the treatment because the client will have more confidence in the change process, feel more responsible for the treatment, and be more invested in it.

It is therefore valuable after each session to reflect with the client on the choices made, the material interaction, the material experience, and the thoughts about the art product. The art product has always proven to be a useful and concrete starting point for discussion and helps the client to distance themselves from the experience during the art work. The formal art elements help to discuss the material interaction and material experience. This allows the art therapist to point out concrete and relevant moments during the session. The observations of the material interaction and material experience during the session help to name concrete moments in the process. The following points can be addressed:

- What did the client do?
- How did the client work? This is about gaining insight into the structuring of the client's art-making. Was there a plan in place that was followed or deviated from? Did an idea develop along the way? How were decisions made? Did the client try different things with the material or not? Did the client need additional guidance? How did the approach work for the client?
- How was the material, technique, and size used perceived? Would the client like to use the material again? Why/why not? Can the client name their own experience or is it difficult? Is what they said congruent with what you observed during the work? Does the client recognize any of the emotions you observed during the work?

- What does the client think about the result? If possible, it may be a good idea to ask other clients to give feedback on the structure and variation of the art product.
- Are there any other discussion points that are relevant at this point?

At the end of the observations, after at least three sessions, an overall reflection can take place. This can be done, for example, by placing all the art products next to each other or hanging them up. The following points may be discussed:

- How did the client work in general during the sessions? Looking back at all the sessions so far, what does the client themself notice? The idea is to gain insight into the client's expressive structuring. Was there usually a plan in place and was it followed or deviated from? Did an idea develop along the way? Did they work differently each time, and if so, what was the reason? How did the client make decisions? Did the client try different things with the material or not? Was it easier one time than the next, and if so, what was the reason? Does the client recognize the way things are designed in situations outside of therapy and does the client name them? Does the client recognize them when you name them? Or does the client see both similarities and differences, and has an idea why?
- How was the material, technique, and format experienced? What are the client's preferences, and can they name the reasons? Can the client name their own experiences or is this difficult? Is there a difference between negative and positive feelings? Does the client recognize this? Does the client recognize the way feelings are acknowledged and expressed in situations outside of therapy? Is what the client is naming congruent with what you have observed in your work?
- How does the client feel about the outcome? Does the client see similarities between the structure and variation of the art products and the way they were designed?
- Looking back at previous sessions, what did the client particularly like or find difficult?
- How does the client see the follow-up? Is there a relationship between the art therapy and the request for help? Does the client have preferences, expectations, desires?
- Does the client see similarities between the art therapy and ways of feeling, acting, and thinking in other situations?

It is up to the art therapist to determine the appropriate time to discuss the relationship between patterns in material interaction, experience, and art product and patterns in thinking, feeling, and acting outside of therapy. Sometimes, the client will draw parallels. But, it can also be considered whether or not the client can recognize the similarities that the art therapist may see. This will probably not be an issue in the first session, but gradually it is relevant to explore whether the client recognizes them. In the final reflection (after at least three sessions), you pay attention to this anyway.

These questions and order are not set in stone. It is up to the therapist's expertise to judge for each client whether and how the reflection can be given a form appropriate to the practical situation. It can be done individually or in a group.

If the client finds it difficult to reflect, which is also important to observe, it may help to have the client look at the art product in the third person. A question might then be, for example:

Suppose these three art products are not yours. Someone else made them and they are hanging here in the hallway. What would you notice? What would it tell you about who made them? Would it tell you anything about the kind of person they are?

Reflecting together provides insight into (1) the client's ability to reflect; (2) the client's ability to recognize and express feelings; (3) the client's preferences; and (4) parallels to situations outside of art therapy. It also contributes to a joint discussion about follow-up: what are the client's expectations and wishes regarding the treatment? Understanding these aspects contributes to the formulation of an art therapy assessment, which is the basis for the indication and choice of interventions. By discussing this with the client, the client becomes coresponsible for his or her own treatment. This strengthens the client's autonomy and generally contributes to the treatment process. This is also called shared decision-making and is an important part of evidence-based practice. Evidence-based practice means that treatment is based not only on the best available scientific evidence but also on a balance between the client's preferences, expectations, and wishes and the professional's (own) expertise.

2.11 Role of the therapeutic relationship

"What can you actually see in my work?" is a question often asked by clients. It shows how vulnerable a client is and can feel. The therapeutic relationship plays an important role in the initiation of change processes within art therapy (Gazit et al., 2021; Hinz, 2020) and in the outcome of treatment (Crits-Christoph et al., 2013; David et al., 2021; Flückiger et al., 2020). And the foundation for this is laid in the observation and assessment phase. It is important that a client trusts the therapist enough to dare to open up to exploration in the art form. Other research (Crits-Christoph et al., 2013; David et al., 2021; Flückiger et al., 2020) also shows the importance of a mutual positive relationship and cooperation between therapist and client and agreement on the purpose of the observation and assessment phase.

It is therefore important from the outset that the client can and dares to trust that the observation and assessment is in the interest of their treatment. This can be done, for example, by being transparent about how the observations are being made. This does not need to be done in detail, as this may trigger the client too much cognitively and thus affect the experience of the work, but a general outline can be given in accordance with the ArTA methodology.

Again, it is important to be able to handle the full range of art material and different structures. For example, in §1.3, it was described that the context of the session plays an important role. Structuring the context of the session, based on instruction, material, technique, and tools, in such a way that it meets the individual needs of the client contributes to basic confidence.

This basic security is needed to challenge the client in the third or later session of the observation phase. The therapist pays full attention to the client (Van Lith, 2020) while at the same time demonstrating sufficient (emotional) support and skill in offering instructions tailored to the client. This requires not only mastery of the therapeutic effects of the art form but also a great deal of insight into psychological processes. Although the concepts of transference and countertransference originated in psychoanalysis, it is a phenomenon that every art therapist has to deal with, regardless of which psychotherapeutic stream they work in, as well as in art therapeutic observation and assessment. It is therefore important that the therapist has sufficient self-observation skills and is aware of the aspects they bring to the therapeutic relationship. These include personal likes and dislikes for certain materials and structures. Personal characteristics such as age, gender, and background also play a role (Talwar, 2015). By being aware of these, the therapist can be fully present in the session and attuned to the client. Unconscious and unintentional provocation of the countertransference is avoided as much as possible.

2.12 Indication

Based on the relationship between patterns of material interaction, material experience, and the art product, the client's balance and adaptability can be assessed. As mentioned earlier, it remains important to formulate this specifically to the uniqueness of each client. Gaining insights into these aspects guides the indication process. The purpose of the formulation of an ArTA assessment is to evaluate if and why art therapy is an appropriate form of treatment for the client[11] and, if so, what direction the treatment should take, what treatment goals can be formulated, and what duration, structure, and frequency of treatment are appropriate.[12] This provides guidance in choosing interventions that will enable the client to work on the treatment goals. It gives direction to the methodical phasing of the treatment, the choice of specific art interventions, and the therapeutic attitude. Art therapy assessment thus forms the basis for clinical reasoning.[13]

The questions that can be asked at the time of indication are:

1 *What are the client's challenges and strengths?*
   You have used ArTA to get a good picture of the client's imbalance and adaptability. How are these characterized? In what direction and to what extent is

there imbalance? How fixed is the pattern of imbalance? What potential for development do you see in the aspects of adaptability? Can you nuance this based on the four sub-aspects of openness, flexibility, self-management, and creativity? For example, do you see that the client shows adaptability in terms of openness but seems to have a bit more difficulty with self-management? Where does this show up? What factors influence this? For example, a client who finds it difficult to sense material experience, may find this easier when working with sensory material, as long as clear instruction is given.

2   *What is the focus of treatment and what are the goals?*
Broadly speaking, ArTA is always about restoring or developing the balance between thinking and feeling and increasing adaptability. Insight into a possible imbalance between thinking and feeling provides starting points for determining the treatment focus to restore the balance. In ArTA, thinking and feeling are seen as two sides of the same coin. For example, if the client has an imbalance toward thinking, treatment will focus on sensing, recognizing, and expressing feelings. The extent and speed with which this is possible depends on how fixed the pattern of imbalance is. In general, the less rigid the pattern, the more adaptability and opportunity for change. Again, it is important to have insight into what is specifically going on with the client in order to formulate realistic and achievable goals that are best tailored to the client's needs, desires, and feasibility. A good understanding of this will help to assess the feasibility of the goals set and the duration, frequency, and interventions of the treatment required to achieve them. In doing so, it is also important to consider the aspects of the setting in which you work. Perhaps you have limited time or a limited number of sessions. Then you will have to realistically adjust the treatments goals accordingly.

3   *What features of art therapy will enable this client to achieve change?*
Section 1.3 discussed how the combination of properties of materials, techniques, and tools and instructions – the so-called mixing panel – can be methodically used to structure the art therapy session in such a way that it allows the client to have specific experiences that contribute to restoring balance and increasing adaptability.

Clients whose imbalance leans toward thinking may benefit from more affective experiences in which feelings can be recognized, acknowledged, and expressed. Clients whose imbalance is toward feeling may benefit from more cognitive experiences in which feelings are appropriately expressed and regulated through cognitive control. Here, the material interaction leading to material experiences provides an opportunity to explore feelings and (other) ways of dealing with them in the here and now.

ArTA, of course, is primarily focused on this methodical use of the art form. But in addition, it may also be important in this step to consider other, perhaps more generic aspects such as group size, and aspects of the therapeutic relationship. Of course, appropriate within the context of the setting in which you work.

4 *What effects do you expect?*

This is also called prognosis and enables the therapist to estimate the duration of the treatment, the frequency of sessions per week, and the form of the session (individual, individual in a group, group). The degree of imbalance and adaptability provide guidance. Usually, the treatment prognosis of a client with extreme and rigid patterns in material interaction, material experience, and art product is less favorable. If more adaptability – openness, flexibility, self-management, and creativity – is observed, the prognosis is usually more favorable.

5 *How can these effects be explained?*

Especially in the communication with the client and other professionals involved in treatment, it can be important to be able to explain the added value of art therapy for this client. What makes art therapy an appropriate form of therapy, specifically for this client? For this, you can use, for example, the theory of neuro-analogous processes described in Section 1.5 which states that the processes underlying (dysfunctional) behavior in everyday situations are analogous to the processes activated during art-making. The experiential nature of art therapy trough the methodical use of the art form distinguishes art therapy form other forms of treatment. Allowing the client to come to a different material interaction and thereby gain different experiences offers an entry point to influence these processes that we know are difficult to reach trough verbal language and cognition. This allows the client to regain balance and adaptability.

6 *Are there other factors at play?*

Consider, for example, the client's age, physical functioning factors, living conditions, and cultural background, but also your own knowledge and skills that you, as a therapist, need to master in order to shape the treatment.

Establishing an indication therefore requires a critical assessment. It may be that the client would benefit more from another form of therapy. Again, try to make a good case for this. If the client is being offered several forms of therapy, it is also important to keep thinking critically about the role of art therapy: what does art therapy add to the other forms of therapy?

I would also like to reiterate the importance of considering the client's wishes, preferences, and expectations. As a professional, you can think and want all sorts of things, but ultimately the client has to change themself. Being transparent about your own ideas about how art therapy can support this can help the client to think along with you and come to agreements together. This is the basis for further collaboration in therapy.

Notes

1 You can download the full English dissertation and all research articles from my website (https://www.ingridpenzes.com/en/publicaties) or https://repository.ubn.ru.nl/bitstream/handle/2066/216188/216188.pdf?sequence=1

2 Client refers to all persons participating in art therapy. Depending on the context (therapy, training, coaching), this can be a patient, student or employee.

3 Art work refers to both the art process (the active *work*) and the art product (the *art work*).

4 Some sources that elaborate on this are: Betts (2006, 2012, 2016), Gilroy et al. (2012), Hogan (2015), Jones (2020), Rubin (2016), Van Hooren et al. (2021) and Van Lith (2016).

5 See also Section 2.5 material experience to read what experience this evokes in this client.

6 To translate these findings into three-dimensional art products, follow-up research will need to take place.

7 The underlying research has shown that training assessors in observing the formal elements has a positive impact on inter-rater reliability.

8 The difference between movement and dynamic can be tricky. They are closely related: a lot of movement is often accompanied by a lot of dynamics. However, there is a relevant difference. Movement is mainly about the amount and direction of movement. Dynamic is mainly about the tension in the image and the vitality of the movement.

9 In this case, colored ink was used that is a fluid material with lots of pigment. This material is difficult to control and easy to mix, so an art product made with this material usually has little contour and more mixture of color.

10 The formal elements do not always reflect all aspects of material interaction. For example, 'shaping' can be difficult to see if layers have been painted on top of each other or if a sketch was first set up with pencil and then worked in with paint. This is one reason why observation of the process as well as the product is important.

11 This may also mean that art therapy is not indicated. In that case, another form of treatment or counseling is more appropriate for achieving the goals.

12 An indication is basically theoretical. In practice, the applicable frameworks within the relevant institution/organization and context must be taken into account. These may be prescriptive with regard to the duration of treatment, frequency, etc., among other things. For example, if the prescribed maximum duration of treatment is shorter than deemed necessary based on the indication, it can be decided to adjust the treatment focus and goals accordingly or, in extreme cases, not to indicate art therapy.

13 The elaboration of this is beyond the purpose of this book.

References

Acton, M. (2009). *Learning to look at paintings* (2nd ed.). Routledge.

Betensky, M.G. (1973). *Self-discovery through self-expression: Use of art psychotherapy with and adolescents*. Charles C. Thomas.

Betts, D.J. (2005). *A systematic analysis of art therapy assessment and rating instrument literature* [PhD dissertation, The Florida State University]. The Florida State University/School of Visual Arts and Dance.

Betts, D.J. (2006). Art therapy assessments and rating instruments: Do they measure up? *The Arts in Psychotherapy, 33*, 422–434. https://doi.org/10.1016/j.aip.2006.08.001

Betts, D.J. (2016). Art therapy assessments: An overview. In D.E. Gussak & M.L. Rosal (Eds.), *The Wiley-Blackwell handbook of art therapy* (pp. 501–513). Wiley-Blackwell.

Betts, D.J. (2012). Positive art therapy assessment: looking towards positive psychology for new directions in the art therapy evaluation process. In A. Gilroy, R. Tipple, & C. Brown (Eds.), *Assessment in art therapy* (pp. 203–218). Routledge.

Betts, D.J., & Groth-Marnat, G. (2014). The intersection of art therapy and psychological assessment: Unified approaches to the use of drawings and artistic processes. In L. Handler & A.D. Thomas (Eds.), *Drawings in assessment and psychotherapy* (pp. 268–285). Routledge.

Boermans, L.A.M., & van der Borght, A. (2017). *Beeldende begrippen. Begrippen in beeldende vormgeving* [Art Concepts. Concepts in the visual art making]. LAMBO.

Buck. J.N. (1948). The H-T-P technique, a qualitative and quantitative scoring manual. *Journal of Clinical psychology Monograph Supplement, 4*, 1–120.

Case, C., & Dalley, T. (2014). *The handbook of art therapy.* Routledge, Taylor and Francis Group.

Chilton, G. (2013). Art therapy and flow: A review of the literature and applications. *Art Therapy: Journal of the American Art Therapy Association, 30*, 64–70. https://doi.org/10.1080/07421656.2013.787211

Claessens, S., Annemans, F., Pénzes, I., & Van Hooren, S. (2016). Meetinstrumenten in de beeldende therapie. Een inventariserend onderzoek naar de kennis en het gebruik van meetinstrumenten [Measuring instruments in art therapy. An inventory study of the knowledge and use of measurement instruments]. *Tijdschrift voor Vaktherapie, 12*(1), 27–34.

Cohen, B.M., Hammer, J., & Singer, S. (1986). The Diagnostic Drawing Series (DDS): A systematic approach to art therapy evaluation and research. *The Arts in Psychotherapy, 5*(1), 11–21.

Cohen, B.M., Mills, A., & Kijak, K. (1994). An introduction to the Diagnostic Drawing Series: A standardized tool for diagnostic and clinical use. *Art therapy, Journal of the American Art Therapy Association, 11*(2), 105–110.

Conrad, S.M., Hunter, H.L., & Krieshok, T.S. (2011). An exploration of the formal elements in adolescents' drawings: General screening for socio-emotional concerns. *The Arts in Psychotherapy, 38*, 340–349.

Crits-Christoph, P., Gibbons, M.B.C., & Mukherjee, D. (2013). Psychotherapy process-outcome research. In: M.J. Lambert (Ed.), *Bergin and Garfield's handbook of psychotherapy and behavior change* (pp. 298–340). Wiley.

Czamanski-Cohen, J., & Weihs, K.L. (2016). The bodymind model: A platform for studying the mechanisms of change induced by art therapy. *The Arts in Psychotherapy, 51*, 63–71. https://doi.org/10.1016/j.aip.2016.08.006

David, I.A.B., Or, M.B., Regev, D., & Snir, C. (2021). Changes over time in therapeutic and art therapy working alliances in simulated art therapy sessions. *The Arts in Psychotherapy, 75*, article 101804. https://doi.org/10.1016/j.aip.2021.101804

De Visser, A. (2010). *Hardop Kijken* [Looking out loud]. SUN.

Eisenbach, N. Snir, S., & Regev, D. (2014). Identification and characterization of symbols emanating from the spontaneous artistic product of victims of childhood trauma who have created art throughout their lives. *The Arts in Psychotherapy, 48*, 45–56. https://doi.org/10.1016/j.aip.2014.12.002

Elbing, U., & Hacking, S. (2001). Nürtinger Beurteilungsskala und Diagnostic Assessment of Psychiatric Art: Neue Wege zur Evaluation der Bilder von Kunsttherapie-patienten [Nuertingen Assessment Scale and Diagnostic Assessment of Psychiatric Art: New Ways to Evaluate Art Therapy Patients' Images]. *Zeitschrift für Musik-, Tanz- und Kunsttherapie, 12*(3), 133–144.

Eytan, L., & Elkis-Abuhoff, D.L. (2013). Indicators of depression and self-efficacy in the PPAT drawings of normative adults. *The Arts in Psychotherapy, 40*, 291–297.

Flückiger, C., Del Re, A.C., Wlodasch, D., Horvath, A.O., Solomonov, N., & Wampold, B.E. (2020). Assessing the alliance – outcome association adjusted for patient characteristics and treatment processes: A meta-analytic summary of direct comparisons. *Journal of Counseling Psychology, 67*(6), 706–711. https://doi.org/10.1037/cou000042

Gale, M. (2016). *Tate modern. The handbook.* Tate.

Gantt, L. (2001). The formal elements art therapy scale: A measurement system for global variables in art. *Art Therapy: Journal of the American Art Therapy Association, 18,* 51–55.

Gantt, L. (2004). The case for formal art therapy assessments. *Art Therapy: Journal of the American Art Therapy Association, 21,* 18–29.

Gantt, L., & Tabone, C. (1998). *The formal elements art therapy scale: The rating manual.* Gargoyle.

Gazit, I., Snir, S., Regev, D., & Bat Or, M. (2021). Relationships between the Therapeutic Alliance and Reactions to Artistic Experience With Art Materials in an Art Therapy Simulation. *Frontiers in Psychology.* https://doi.org/10.3389/fpsyg.2021.560957

Gerrits, A. (Ed.). (2018). *KPC-model: beschouwingswijzer voor beeldende kunst.* [KPC model: contemplation guide for the visual arts]. Kunstcontext.

Gilroy, A., & McNeilly, G. (2000). *The changing shape of art therapy: New developments in theory and practice.* Jessica Kingsley.

Gilroy, A., Tipple, R., & Brown, C. (2012). *Assessment in art therapy.* Routledge.

Gussak, D., & Rosal, M. (Eds.). (2016). *The Wiley handbook of art therapy.* Wiley-Blackwell.

Hacking, S. (1999). *The psychopathology of everyday art: A quantitative study* [PhD dissertation, University of Keele]. University of Keele.

Haeyen, S. (2018). *Effects of art therapy. The case of personality disorders cluster B/C* [PhD dissertation, Radboud University Nijmegen]. Behavioural Science Institute. 183225.pdf (ru.nl)

Hilbuch, A., Snir, S., Regev, D., & Orkibi, H. (2016). The role of art materials in the transferential relationship: Art psychotherapists' perspective. *The Arts in Psychotherapy, 49,* 19–26. https://doi.org/10.1016/j.aip.2016.05.011

Hinz, L.D. (2009). *Expressive therapies continuum.* Routledge.

Hinz, L.D. (2015). Expressive therapies continuum: Use and value demonstrated with case study. *Canadian Art Therapy Association Journal, 28,* 43–50.

Hinz, L.D. (2020). *Expressive therapies continuum: A framework for using art in therapy* (2nd ed.). Routledge Taylor & Francis.

Hogan, S. (2015). *Art therapy theories. A critical introduction.* Taylor & Francis.

Huntsman, P. (2016). *Thinking about art. A thematic guide to art history.* Wiley Blackwell/Association of Art Historians.

Joiner, T.E., Schmidt, K.L., & Barnett, J. (1996). Size, detail, and line heaviness in children's drawings as correlates of emotional distress; (more) negative evidence. *Journal of Personality Assessment, 67,* 127–141.

Jones, P. (2020). *The arts therapies. A revolution in health care.* Routledge. https://doi.org/10.4324/9781315536989

Kagin, S.L., & Lusebrink, V.B. (1978). The expressive therapies continuum. *Art Psychotherapy, 5,* 171–180.

Kaplan, F.F. (2012). Art-based assessments. In C.A. Malchiodi (Ed.), *Handbook of art therapy* (pp. 25–35). The Guilford Press.

Kim, S., Kang, H., Chung, S., & Hong, E. (2012). A statistical approach to comparing the effectiveness of several art therapy tools in estimating the level of a psychological state. *The Arts in Psychotherapy, 39*, 397–403.

Kramer, E. (1975). The problem of quality in art. In E. Ulman & P. Dachinger (Eds.), *Art therapy in theory and practice* (pp. 43–59). Schocken.

Lowenfeld, V. (1952). *Creative and mental growth* (2nd ed.). Macmillan.

Lusebrink, V.B. (2010). Assessment and therapeutic application of the expressive therapies continuum: Implication for brain structures and functions. *Art Therapy: Journal of the American Art Therapy Association, 27*(4), 168–177. https://doi.org/10.1080/07 421656.2010.10129380

Mattson, D.C. (2009). Accessible image analysis for art assessment. *The Arts in Psychotherapy, 36*, 208–213.

Murray, H.A. (1943). *Thematic apperception test*. Harvard University.

Nan, J.K., & Hinz, L.D. (2012). Applying the fFormal Elements Art Therapy Scale (FEATS) to adult in an asian population. *Art Therapy: Journal of the American Art Therapy Association, 29*(3), 127–132.

Naumburg, M. (1966). *Dynamically oriented art therapy*. Grune & Stratton.

Naumburg, M. (2001). Spontaneous art in education and psychotherapy. *Art Therapy: American Journal of Art Therapy, 40*(1), 46–64.

Panofsky, E. (1932). Zum Problem der Beschreibung und Inhaltsdeutung von Werken der bildenden Kunst [On the problem of description and content interpretation of works of fine art]. *Logos, 21*, 103–119.

Panofsky, E. (1939). *Studies in iconology: Humanistic themes in the art of the renaissance*. Oxford.

Pénzes, I. (2020). *Art form and mental health. Studies on art therapy observation and assessment in adult mental health* [PhD dissertation, Radboud University Nijmegen]. Behavioral Science Institute. https://repository.ubn.ru.nl/bitstream/handle/2066/216188/216188.pdf?sequence=1

Pénzes, I., van Hooren, S., Dokter, D., Smeijsters, H., & Hutschemaekers, G. (2018). How art therapists observe mental health using formal elements in art products: Structure and variation as indicators for balance and adaptability. *Frontiers in Psychology/Clinical and Health psychology*. https://doi.org/10.3389/fpyg.2018.01611

Rankanen, M. (2016). *The visible spectrum: Participant's experiences of the process and impacts of art therapy* [PhD dissertation, Aalto University]. Aalto University.

Rhyne, J. (1973). *The Gestalt art therapy experience*. Brooks/Cole.

Rubin, J.A. (2009). *Introduction to art therapy. Sources and resources*. Routledge Taylor Francis.

Rubin, J.A. (2016). *Approaches to art of art therapy, theory and technique*. Taylor Francis. https://doi.org/10.4324/9781315716015

Schaverien, J. (1999). Art within analysis: Scapegoat, transference and transformation. *Journal of Analytic Psychology, 44*(4), 479–510. https://doi.org/10.1111/1465-5922.00116

Schaverien, J. (2005). Art and active imagination: reflections on transference and the image. *International Journal of Art Therapy, 10*(2), 39–52. https://doi.org/10.1080/17454830500345959

Schoch, K., Ostermann, T., & Gruber, H. (2017). Measuring art: Methodical development of a quantitative rating instrument measuring pictorial expression (RizbA). *The Arts in Psychotherapy, 55*, 73–79.

Simon, R.M. (2001). The significance of pictorial styles in art therapy. *Art Therapy: American Journal of Art Therapy, 40*(1), 92–108.

Springham, N., Findlay, D., Woods, A., & Harris, J. (2012). How can art therapy contribute to mentalization in borderline personality disorder? *International Journal of Art Therapy, 17*, 115–129. https://doi.org/10.1080/17454832.2012.734835

Stuhler-Bauer, A., & Elbing, U. (2003). Die Phänomenologische Bilderfassung: Ein Kunsttherapeutisches Instrument [The phenomenological image capture: An art therapy tool]. *Zeitschrift für Musik-, Tanz- und Kunsttherapie, 14*(1), 32–46.

Talwar, S. (2015). Culture, diversity, and identity: From margins to center. *Art Therapy: Journal of the American Art Therapy Association, 32*(3), 100–103. https://doi.org/10.1080/07421656.2015.1060563

Taylor, J.C. (2014). *Learning to look. A handbook for the visual arts* (2nd ed.). The University of Chicago Press.

Thomas, K., & Cody, M. (2012). Three Starting Points (3SP): An art-based assessment method. In A. Gilroy, R. Tipple, & C. Brown (Eds.), *Assessment in art therapy* (pp. 153–168). Routledge.

Thyme, K.E., Wiberg, B., Lundman, B., & Graneheim, U.H. (2013). Qualitative content analysis in art psychotherapy research: Concepts, procedures, and measures to reveal the latent meaning in pictures and the words attached to the pictures. *The Arts in Psychotherapy, 40*, 101–107.

Ulman, E., & Bernard, I.L. (2001). An experimental approach to the judgement of psychopathology from paintings. *Art Therapy: American Journal of Art Therapy, 40*, 82–91.

Van der Kamp, M.T., Cuijpers, W., & van de Vlies, A.M. (2012). *ILO-UvA: Begrippen voor kunstanalyse* [*Concepts for art analysis*]. University of Amsterdam.

Van Hooren, S.A.H., van Busschbach, J., Waterink, W., & Abbing, A. (2021). Werkingsmechanismen van vaktherapie: Naar een onderbouwing en verklaring van effecten – work in progress [Working mechanisms of arts therapies: Towards a foundation and explanation of effects – work in progress]. *Tijdschrift voor Vaktherapie, 17*(2), 4–12.

Van Lith, T. (2016). Art therapy in mental health: A systematic review of approaches and practices. *The Arts in psychotherapy, 47*(2), 9–22. http://dx.doi.org/10.1016/j.aip.2015.09.003

Van Lith, T. (2020). Fostering client voice and choice through art therapy. *Art Therapy Journal of the American Art Therapy Association, 37*(4), 167–168. https://doi.org//10.1080/07421656.2020.1847577

Wadeson, H. (1980). *Art psychotherapy*. John Wiley & Sons.

Wadeson, H. (2002). The anti-assessment devil's advocate. *Art Therapy: Journal of the American Art Therapy Association, 19*(4), 168–170.

Wilson, S., & Lack, J. (2016). *Tate guide to modern art terms*. Tate.

Chapter 3

ArTA

The methodical application

Introduction

In Chapter 1, the basic conceptual framework of ArTA was described. And in Chapter 2, the underlying theory was described, and we saw that the goal of art therapy observation and assessment is to gain insight into the client's mental health. This chapter describes the methodical application of ArTA, in particular the four steps of observing, analyzing, interpreting, and formulating. These steps build from the observation of material interaction, material experience, and art product to the analysis of patterns and their interpretation in terms of balance and adaptability as aspects of mental health. On this basis, an art therapist can assess whether and to what extent there is an imbalance between thinking and feeling and the client's adaptability, specified by self-management, openness, flexibility, and creativity. Also, information can be given about the client's ability to reflect and their own wishes and preferences which are important to include in the context of shared decision-making. This helps the art therapist to evaluate whether the client could benefit from art therapy. It supports the formulation of treatment goals and the selection of art interventions that contribute to their achievement. But how does one do this in clinical practice? That is what this chapter is about: the concrete application. You will be introduced to the four steps of ArTA in which you work from observation to assessment. It is important to emphasize that this is not a "cookbook," as the method cannot be applied without professional art therapy training and expertise. On paper, we separate these steps. In practice, these steps will flow smoothly into each other.

3.1   The ArTA observation form

The ArTA observation form is primarily a tool for learning and applying ArTA in practice. For example, I use it in the ArTA Basic Course to allow participating art therapists to practice using ArTA with their own clients. And as with so much of what you are learning that is new, it takes a little extra time in the beginning. Once you know how to systematically and purposefully observe material

DOI: 10.4324/9781003428305-3

interaction, material experience, and the art product, how they are related, and how to interpret them in terms of balance and adaptability, you will not need to fill it out so extensively for every client. You can then shorten the ArTA observation form. You can do this, for example, by not filling in all the material interaction categories, but simply placing the material interaction style for each session on the affective-rational continuum. Or by noting the degree of structure and variation for each session rather than filling in all the formal elements. Filling in only the patterns across sessions might be another shortcut.

Ultimately, it is about being able to formulate the direction and degree of imbalance and the degree of adaptability. And that based on this, you can evaluate whether the client could benefit from art therapy and why (or why not). And if so, what treatment goals are appropriate and achievable. The last part of the ArTA observation form provides guidance and can be used to help communicate with the client and others involved in the treatment. Based on your own experience and expertise, you will be able to tailor this to be specific and appropriate to your own place of work.

Using ArTA, you can determine which interventions will give the client the best opportunity to work on the stated goals. Within ArTA, we use the art therapy mixing panel (see §1.3 and the indication (see §2.12) for this purpose in which we assume analogous processes (see §1.5).

Chapter 1 described how ArTA assumes that we can relate the coherence of patterns of material interaction, material experience, and art product to the degree of imbalance and adaptability, but that it is especially important to pay attention to the uniqueness of the client. The specification and nuanced formulation of these characteristics on the ArTA observation form does not only do justice to the uniqueness of the client. It also provides insight into possible entry points for treatment.

Art therapy is experiential; by interacting with the art form, a person can feel bodily signals and related emotions in the here and now. Especially when a client has difficulty recognizing, acknowledging, or expressing emotions, the therapist can first offer the art form in a way that allows a person to experience relaxation, playfulness, and other positive emotions and to dare to acknowledge them. From there, the client can experience that it is not necessary to avoid emotions, and space is created to experience and redirect negative emotions as well.

For example, experiencing different materials may provide an entry point to feel what is preferred if it is noted that the client has difficulty with self-management but is open to new experiences. This can contribute to making choices and thus increasing self-management. Or, if a client is found to have an imbalance in thinking, and this is particularly evident in the way they move when interacting with materials, then an intervention can be aimed at getting the client to move in a different way, step by step. This can help the client to become aware and possibly conscious of the accompanying physical sensations and feelings, thus creating more balance between thinking and feeling.

3.2   The four steps of ArTA

ArTA consists of four steps: observing, analyzing, interpreting, and formulating (see Figure 3.1). They progress from observing material interaction, material experience, and art product per session, to analyzing patterns and their correlation across sessions, to interpreting them in terms of balance and adaptability, and to formulating and describing these aspects. In practice, these steps flow into each other. We separate them here for convenience. Each step is explained in detail below.

3.2.1 Step 1: Observing

The first step is observing. In this step, material interaction, material experience, and the art product are observed per session, for at least three sessions. As described in Chapter 1, observation is about observing as objectively and systematically as possible. In this step, you are not yet concerned with the meaning of your observations. You observe the style of material interaction, the striking aspects of material experience, and the structure and variation based on formal art elements in each art product. Always keep the context of the art-making process in the session in mind.

3.2.1.1 Context of the session

Before you start observing, it is important to be able to place your observations in the context of the session. Chapter 1 described how the characteristics of the used materials, techniques and tools, and instructions determine the structure of an art-making process. In Chapter 2, it became clear that this affects the observation of material interaction, material experience, and the art product. Therefore, space has been made for this at the top of the observation form. You note:

• What material, technique, and tool were used. You will also note whether this was given by the therapist or chosen by the client. This will be important later when observing, analyzing, and interpreting your observations.
• The format of the paper the client worked on. This is especially important when later analyzing and interpreting the formal elements of the art product. For example, you can determine whether the movement was large or small.

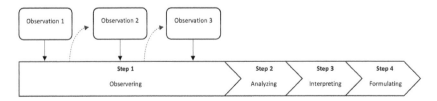

Figure 3.1 The four steps of ArTA.

- The instructions you gave as the therapist. This, in addition to the characteristics of the material and technique used, may influence the degree of structure the client needed to start an art-making process. The instruction may also influence the material interaction, the material experience, and the art product.

You can then begin to write down your observations. It is a good idea to write down these observations and what came up in reflection as soon as possible after the session so that everything is fresh in your mind. The art product is kept, so you can take time to do this later if necessary, but preferably before the next session.

3.2.1.2 Material interaction

In terms of material interaction, after each session, note your main observations by category: movement, pressure, grip, organization, tempo, physical contact, rhythm, space, lining, mixing of color, shaping, and dialogue (see §2.4). To do this, it is important to know what is meant by each of these 12 categories (see Table 2.2). It is advisable to do this as succinctly as possible, using keywords, for example, as this will help you to extract the essence of what you have observed. Many categories include a gradation, such as large or small movement, a lot or little force, etc. These are printed in italics on the observation form and can help you focus your observations. You may not have made any salient observations in all 12 categories, in which case you should fill in those categories as well (for example, "no salient observations").

These categories will then help you determine the style of material interaction. As you read in Chapter 2 (see §2.4), this involves combining the different categories. Based on this combination, the style of material interaction can be placed on a continuum from rational to affective. These are briefly summarized in Table 2.3. In practice, clients usually do not have a completely rational or affective style of material interaction. A continuum means that a client's style can be positioned somewhere along the line. In this step, it is particularly important whether you find the style of material interaction to be more rational or more affective. You briefly describe this on the observation form for each session. The thick short vertical arrows on the observation form indicate this.

3.2.1.3 Material experience

Observations of material experience are briefly described on the observation form for each session. There are no categories for material experience, as there are for material interaction, into which you can classify your observations. What is important is that you observe what emotions, if any, the client is feeling, recognizing, allowing, expressing, and regulating (see §2.5). For example, a client may not recognize feelings at all, may be unable or afraid to allow them, may be overwhelmed by them, etc. There may also be a difference between negative and positive feelings. You can pay attention to the client's facial expressions, posture, and verbal expressions in relation to the material being worked with. Because it can be very difficult to observe the client's inner experience "from the outside," it is always advisable to bring it up during reflection. Even if you have not observed any experience, it is important to note it and reflect on it with the client. In this way, the client can indicate how the material was experienced and what factors may have influenced it (material that was difficult to control, the therapist's technique and instructions that may or may not have provided structure, etc.).

3.2.1.4 Art product

For the art product, fill in the formal elements for each product: movement, dynamic, contour, repetition, mixture of color, and color saturation (see §2.6). It is important that you know what is meant by each formal element (see Table 2.4). Consider the size of the art product and the materials used. As you read in §2.6, the individual formal elements have no diagnostic value. The combination is important: it determines the degree of structure and variation of the art product. This is indicated in the observation form by the thick short vertical arrows.

Structure can be placed on a continuum from high to low (see Figure 2.1 in §2.6.2). In determining this, it is recommended first to look at the combination of movement, dynamic, and contour. These are the primary formal elements that, in combination, strongly define the structure. Little movement and little dynamic combined with a lot of contour results in a high structure; a lot of movement and dynamic combined with little contour results in low structure. You then observe the other formal elements to determine whether they strengthen or weaken the structure.

As for variation, this step is about determining the degree per art product. You can observe variation in the diversity of the formal elements. For example, the presence of variation in contour, as some parts are clearly outlined and other parts are less or not. Or variation in movement, in which there are both small and larger movements, in different directions. This is usually strongly related to the extent to which the client has engaged in dialogue in the material interaction and tried out different properties of the material. On the observation form, note the degree of variation you see in the art product, with a brief explanation if necessary.

Section 2.9 briefly addressed the situation where an art product is not completed within a session. If the client chooses to continue working on this art product in a second session, the observation of the art product can take place after the second session. It is important to note this on the observation form. It provides relevant information about, for example, the pace at which the work was done, the importance the client attached to the end result, and so on. The case study in Chapter 4 also deals with this. Of course, the opposite is also possible: the client creates several art products in one session. Even then, it is important to note this because it provides relevant information about the pace of the work and the importance the client attaches to the end result. It is up to the expertise of the art therapist to decide whether or not to observe multiple art products within a session. It may also be decided to note the most typical image. However, it is by no means the case that the observation of several art products in one session completes the observation. In fact, it is interesting to observe whether or not the client does this again during the minimum of three sessions and what factors (material, technique, instruction) might be involved.

3.2.1.5 Reflection

Whether and how you reflect with the client after each session depends, among other things, on the client's ability to do so (see also §2.10). It is always a good idea to reflect briefly with the client at the end of the session. The main goal is to include the client's own perspective in the art therapy observation and assessment. Even if you do not have a specific discussion about the session, what the client says about the process of art-making and/or the art product can be valuable to note. Another goal is to gain insight into the client's ability to reflect. If this proves difficult due to personal characteristics or state of mind, you can be more directive in your reflections. Rather than asking open-ended questions, you may want to list some of your own observations and assess whether or not the client acknowledges them. Section 2.10 provides some guidelines for items to reflect upon together after each session. On the observation form, note what you notice about the client's reflectiveness and perspective.

3.2.2 Step 2: Analyzing

The second step is analyzing. Based on the observations from the three observation sessions, you will see what patterns emerge in material interaction, material experience, and the structure and variation of art products. Thus, this step takes place after you have completed at least three observation sessions. It is possible that after two sessions you already have a good impression of the patterns in material interaction, material experience, and structure and variation of the art product. This impression will also guide your choice of materials for the third observation session. In this session, because you have more control over the context of the session (through material selection, technique, and instruction), you can see if the client can achieve different material interactions and experiences, and changes in structure and variation. This allows you to assess how fixed patterns may be. It is important to analyze the commonalities (what comes up again and again, regardless of the material) as well as the nuances. For example, if it turns out that the client with a pattern of interacting rationally with the material still had moments of dialoguing with the material, and/or there were moments when feelings were expressed, etc., it is valuable to try to identify these. It is then helpful to try to identify what might have influenced this in the context, such as the material used and the instructions given. This is important because it allows you to determine how fixed certain patterns are and thus how much room there is for development/change. This influences the indication.

3.2.2.1 Material interaction

In Step 1, based on the combination of material interaction categories for each session, you identified and positioned the material interaction style on a continuum from rational to affective. In this step, you will analyze the consistency across the three sessions. This is indicated by the horizontal arrow across the three sessions on the observation form. Questions to ask yourself are: What repeats, what comes up again and again? Is it consistent even when the context is different? Are there aspects that are not consistent? What role might the context play? Based on your analysis, describe the pattern of material interaction that is characteristic of this client. In Section 2.4.2, we saw that there are usually three patterns. Write these down on the observation form and explain them briefly.

3.2.2.2 Material experience

In Step 1, you described the material experience for each session. In this step, you will analyze the consistency across the three sessions. This is indicated by the horizontal arrow across the three sessions on the observation form. Questions to ask yourself are: What experiences did you observe during the work? Does the client acknowledge these feelings? Can the client acknowledge and express these feelings or is it difficult? Is the client in control of their feelings or are they overwhelmed by them? What repeats, what comes up again and again? Is it consistent even when the context is different, such as different materials used, or instructions given? Based on your analysis, describe the pattern of material experience that is characteristic of this client. Record this on the observation form.

3.2.2.3 Art product

In Step 1, you determined the degree of structure and variation for each art product based on the combination of formal art elements. In this step, you will analyze the consistency of the art products. This is indicated by the horizontal arrow across the three sessions on the observation form. Consider the context in which the art products were created (possible influence of materials, technique, and instruction). Questions you might ask yourself here are: How much structure and variation do the different products have? Is this the same for all art products, regardless of context? Or are there differences, and how might the context of the session have influenced this? Based on your analysis, describe the pattern of structure and the pattern of variation. Write this down on the observation form.

3.2.2.4 Overall reflection

In Step 1, you may have reflected briefly with the client after each session. After the last session, it is valuable to reflect with the client on the previous sessions (see also §2.10). It is advisable to arrange the art products in chronological order. This can help the client to see what recurs, but also where there may be differences. It provides a starting point for discussing what factors may have influenced this. This reflection is also a time to explore (if this has not been done in previous reflections) the similarities between art work in therapy and thinking, feeling, and acting in situations outside of therapy. In this reflection, it is also important to talk with the client about expectations and wishes for follow-up (treatment). Section 2.10 provides several points to discuss.

You write down the most important findings on the observation form. You describe your impression of the client's ability to reflect, paying particular attention to the client's own perspective, whether the client sees similarities and differences between the work in art therapy, the situation outside of therapy, and the request for help. You also note what expectations, wishes, and preferences there may be regarding follow-up treatment.

3.2.3 Step 3: Interpreting

The third step is interpreting. This is a step that you do not write down directly on the observation form, but which consists mainly of putting the puzzle together. You look at the connection between patterns of material interaction, material experience, and the structure and variation of the art products (see also §2.7). You interpret these in terms of balance and adaptability as aspects of mental health (see also §2.8). In this step, you determine from the patterns whether the client has an imbalance and, if so, in which direction it tends: toward thinking or toward feeling. You also determine the degree of imbalance and the degree of adaptability. Both are explained below. In practice, this will go hand in hand and culminate almost naturally in Step 4, Formulate.

3.2.3.1 Determine the direction of imbalance

There is usually an imbalance with clients: either thinking or feeling takes over and interferes with daily functioning. Observing patterns in material interaction, material experience, and art product provides insight into the direction and degree of imbalance.

For clients with a rational pattern of material interaction, the balance will tilt toward thinking – they will tend to approach situations from the head. A rational pattern of material interaction is characterized by, among other things, thought-fulness, precision, conscientiousness, need for control, and focus on the result, which usually involves a (well-thought-out) plan. The way the client handles art material is analogous to the way the client handles situations outside of therapy. Cognitive control – thinking, planning, organizing – predominates. This is usu-ally reflected in patterns in the structure of the art created. The art products of clients with a rational pattern of material interaction tend to have a combination of less movement and dynamic and more contour. This creates more structure in the art products.

There may be several reasons why clients tilt their balance toward thinking. They may want to avoid (negative) feelings and have difficulty acknowledging, expressing, and/or accepting them. Observing patterns in material experiences is very valuable here. It gives insight into what the client is feeling while expressing, whether the client can admit these feelings, and how the client deals with them.

For clients with an affective pattern of material interaction, the balance will tilt toward feeling. Clients may be overwhelmed by sensations and feelings and have no control over them. One of the characteristics of an affective pattern of material interaction is that it is action oriented. Doing itself is central where im-pulse or feeling is often the cause and/or predominant and where there is usually no well-thought-out plan.

Again, the way the client deals with art material is analogous to the way the client deals with situations outside of therapy. This is usually reflected in patterns in the structure of the art products. The art products of clients with an affective pattern of material interaction tend to have a combination of more movement and dynamic and less contour. This results in less structure in the art products.

There may be several reasons why clients' balance is tilted toward feeling. Perhaps feelings and sensations are so strong that they eliminate cognitive con-trol. Observing patterns in material experiences is very valuable here. Those moments when the client seems to have a little more control are especially valu-able for gaining insight into what the client needs in order to gain a little more control. This may be material, instruction, or something else.

There may also be an alternating pattern of material interaction. This does not mean that both rational and affective aspects can be seen in the material interac-tion, material experience, and structure and variation of the art product, but that there is an alternation between a clear, predominantly rational style of material interaction with a high degree of structure and little variation and a clear, pre-dominantly affective style of material interaction with a low degree of structure and little variation.

There may be several reasons why a client's balance may alternate (extremely) between feeling and thinking. It is possible that the client is trying to avoid or suppress feelings to an extreme degree, and they are completely overwhelming the client when this fails. It is then very valuable to look at the influence of the structure of the context; what activates thinking and what activates feeling?

You note on the observation form if there is an imbalance and how the client's patterns are characterized.

3.2.3.2 Determine the degree of imbalance and adaptability

The less you can place the pattern of material interaction at the ends of the continuum, the less pronounced/extreme the structure of the art products will be, and the more variation in the art products will be observed. This usually means that there is more adaptability and opportunity for change.

The more you can see the pattern of material interaction at one end of the continuum, the more fixed and rigid that pattern usually is. This can also be seen in the structure of the art product. The more extreme the structure is organized or chaotic, the more rigid the pattern tends to be.

Again, you are always looking for where there is an opportunity for change. In fact, art therapists are very good at this. They can do this by looking at the dialogue of material interaction and the degree of variation in the art products. Was the client able to interact with a particular material during the three sessions? When did this happen? We also look at the variation in the art products. You look to see if something more or something different was tried with the material.

After all, variation is associated with play and exploration, but also with making choices. These are aspects that emerge strongly when one pays special attention to the dialogue when observing material interaction: the extent to which the client explores different possibilities and adapts to the properties of the art material. These aspects are related to adaptability.

By observing the variation across three art products, you can see if the client is open to new or different perspectives, is curious, dares to take risks, does not see mistakes as catastrophes, and dares to experiment in unfamiliar situations.

It says something about creativity: the ability to depart from familiar paths, to create something new, and to solve problems. It also shows the client has the flexibility to respond in different ways to different challenges, tasks, people, or situations, or, in this case, art material. This requires the ability to switch between cognitive control and allowing and expressing feelings and acting on them.

It also suggests something of self-management: the ability to make choices by occasionally stepping back and reflecting. Being aware of and paying attention to what is happening in the here and now. Intermediate and concluding reflections with the client provide additional information in this regard (see §2.10).

You note on the observation form your assessment of the extent to which there are fixed patterns leading to the client's imbalance. And your main findings about the client's adaptability and related potential for development.

3.2.4 Step 4: Formulating

The fourth step is formulating. Based on the findings of Steps 1 through 3, you formulate a reasoned description of balance, adaptability (specified by openness, flexibility, creativity, and self-management), reflective capacity, and the client's perspective and indication.

For balance between thinking and feeling, indicate the direction in which the client's imbalance tends and your assessment of the degree of imbalance. Also indicate what is specific to this client and how this relates to situations outside of therapy. Provide a brief rationale and include any input from the client.

For adaptability, indicate where and how much room there is for change in the client. Specify this in terms of openness, creativity, flexibility, and self-management (see Step 3). Also indicate if certain factors influence this, for example, if the client shows more flexibility when the situation is clearly structured by material, technique, and instruction.

For reflective capacity, briefly describe the client's reflective capacity and the key findings from the reflections. Also indicate how the art therapy observations correspond to how the client handles situations outside of therapy. Include the client's perspective on art therapy and possible follow-up treatment. Include the client's preferences, wishes, and expectations in the discussion (shared decision-making).

In the case of an indication, formulate what the above means for follow-up treatment. Based on the direction and degree of imbalance and adaptability, you can assess:

1   Whether and why the client would benefit from art therapy.
2   If so, what the focus and duration of treatment might be to restore balance and increase adaptability. And what treatment goals would fit with that.
3   What art therapy interventions would be appropriate and why.

Now that we have an understanding of the underlying theory and the four steps of ArTA, we move on to the application in clinical practice. The next chapter gives an example of how to apply it in practice. Let's meet Yasper.

Chapter 4

ArTA

A case description

Introduction

To translate the methodical application of ArTA to clinical practice, this chapter uses a case description. We are introduced to Yasper, a fictional name for a client from actual clinical practice. The various sessions and the four steps of observing, analyzing, interpreting, and formulating are described in detail. The use of the ArTA observation form is linked to this, which brings ArTA to life. It gives an impression of what the methodical application of ArTA can look like in clinical practice. It illustrates the relationship between the patterns of material interaction, material experience, and art product within the art form, as well as balance and adaptability as aspects of the client's mental health.

Yasper was introduced to art therapy and the art therapist before the first session. During this meeting, which took place in the art therapy room, it was briefly discussed what art therapy is and what the client's expectations of this form of therapy were in relation to his request for help. The art therapist explained that art therapy is not about creating a beautiful piece of art. That it is not primarily what you make, but how you make it, and that there is no right or wrong. That the way you do it can give insight into where you are stuck, but also where there are opportunities for change. And that on that basis you can look together at how best to achieve that change. The therapist explained that the first few sessions would be used for assessment, working with different materials. And that some materials provide more structure than others, such as a marker versus water color.

The therapist also explained that art therapy was offered in a group of eight clients, with each person working once a week in an individual process and once a week in a group assignment. And that the sessions lasted 75 minutes, including working time, reflection, and cleaning up.

Yasper said that he had not worked with art materials since high school. He apologized in advance if the work was not beautiful, but that he would do his best. He clearly indicated that he was ready for a change, but was not sure how, but was curious to see what art therapy could offer him.

DOI: 10.4324/9781003428305-4

4.1   Case

Yasper is a 37-year-old man. Due to depressive symptoms, he began art therapy as part of a short-term inpatient treatment program. His childhood and adolescence were marked by conformity and perfectionism. He is a widower and father of 6-year-old twin daughters. Depressive symptoms began after his first partner became pregnant. After the birth of their daughters, he started working part-time because his wife wanted to work full time. There was a lot of tension in the relationship during this time. Finally, he decided to get a divorce. At the same time, his wife became seriously ill. He cared for her around the clock with little to no support from family or friends. She died after a long illness. He has had a new partner for a year. However, his symptoms are becoming stronger, and he needs treatment. During the initial consultation, Yasper seemed very friendly, but also tense and insecure. He said he was angry about the way his life has turned out.

4.2   Observations during observation session 1

First, the therapist looked at the materials cabinet with Yasper so that Yasper knew what 2D materials to choose from. There were different types of pencils, markers, colored pencils, crayons, charcoal, pastels, oil pastels, acrylics, watercolors, and colored ink. The therapist explained these materials very briefly, focusing on their properties and possibilities. The therapist then asked Yasper to choose a material and get started.

However, Yasper's eye fell on a book on East Indian ink with Japanese-looking prints that appealed to him. He asked if he could use that as an example. The therapist suggested using colored ink and handed him a sheet of watercolor paper (they agreed on a size of 30 × 42 cm/12 × 16 inches). The therapist also

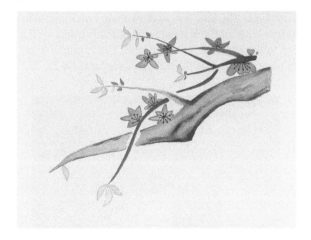

Image 4.1 Art product in observation session 1.

instructed him to tape the sheet of paper to a large board to prevent it from bulging and to allow him to turn the work as he works. The therapist also explained that colored ink won't come out of his clothes, so it might be wise to put on a painting apron. Next, Yasper started to work (see Image 4.1).

He began by placing the large branch diagonally on the paper. He did this slowly and deliberately, holding the brush firmly and from the wrist. He made short, sketchy movements. When he drew the large branch, he left a space for the other branch, even though this was not the case in the example: the branches ran under and over each other. He then worked on this main branch, trying very carefully to reproduce the nuances of color as in the example. He worked with concentration and made minimal contact with his surroundings: all his focus was on his work.

Then the session was over. During the brief reflection, he indicated that he really liked the print from the book. He also liked working from an example but also found it difficult to reproduce it exactly. When the therapist said that colored ink is difficult to control, Yasper sighed: "Yes, quite tiring," yet he really wanted to finish it.

After this session, the therapist filled in the ArTA observation form with the context of the session, the material interaction, the material experience, and the reflection of this first session. And determined the structure and variation of the art product based on the formal elements of movement, dynamic, contour, repetition, mixture of color, and color saturation (see Table 4.1).

4.3   Observations during observation session 2

In the second session, Yasper worked on a group task where all clients were given the same task. He worked on thick paper of 35 × 50 cm/14 × 20 inches on which the therapist had previously taped a frame of 25 × 50 cm/10 × 20 inches with crepe tape. The task was to draw their own initials (first letter of the first name and first letter of the last name) inside this frame with a pencil and to extend the lines to the edges of the crepe tape. The resulting areas were worked in with acrylic paint in colors of their choice (see Image 4.2).

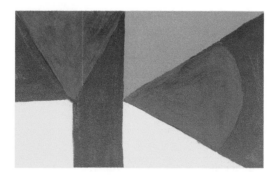

Image 4.2 Art product in observation session 2.

Yasper applied the initials thinly with a pencil. Then, he took a ruler and drew the straight lines a little thicker. Then, he asked if he could draw another line to make a large area smaller (this would be the curved line). He chose four colors from the paint pot: blue, yellow, vermilion, and moss green. First, he put a dot in each area with the color that should go there. Then he worked in the areas. He worked slowly and with concentration, trying to stay clearly within the lines. With short movements, he first painted the contours of the planes, then filled them in at a slightly faster pace. He held the brush firmly. The therapist suggested that he could use a larger brush or paintbrush to fill in the areas. He liked the idea and did so. He worked calmly and with concentration. He seemed to take in what was going on around him. For example, the client next to him wanted to make a color transition in an area. The therapist showed on a separate sheet how to mix the colors and make them more fluid with water. Yasper watched but then continued to work in the same way.

During the brief reflection, Yasper said that he liked acrylics. When the therapist asked why, he said that they were a bit easier to control. The therapist asked how he worked today. He said that he liked to be given a task: "Nice and clear." The therapist asked a bit more about his approach and mentioned that she saw, for example, that before he started painting he first put a dot in each plane. Yasper agreed and explained that he first figured out where to put which color to prevent two adjacent planes from being the same color. When the therapist asked how he came up with the colors, he said that these pots were already together and he thought they would go well together. The therapist asked the group if they noticed anything about the picture. A fellow client said that she noticed how precise it was: "I could never do that so precisely." The therapist asked Yasper if he felt that way. He indicated that he had indeed tried to stay within the lines as much as possible. When the therapist asked him how that went, he said that it went quite easily on the sides where the tape was (pointing to the green area where the paper was torn a bit when the tape was removed, which he regretted), but that he really had to keep his head on the other lines. When the therapist asked if he considered changing his plan while working, he said that he did not. He did say that he really liked his neighbor's color transitions, but that he probably wouldn't be able to do it anyway and would rather continue on the same path.

After this session, the therapist filled in the ArTA observation form with the context of the session, the material interaction, the material experience, and the reflection of this second session. And, again, determined the structure and variation of the art product based on the formal elements of movement, dynamic, contour, repetition, mixture of color, and color saturation (see Table 4.1).

4.4   Observations during session 3: accompanying observation session 1

Yasper was eager to finish the art product from the first session (see Image 4.1). Since the therapist found it very good that he indicated this and did not immediately comply with the request to choose another material, she let him finish the work. Yasper continued to work, starting with the other thinner branches. He worked slowly and the lines were created by letting short movements follow one another. He worked from a steady wrist and held the brush firmly. Then, he added the flowers and leaves. Here, he differed from the example. In the example, the flowers were more random spots where chance has determined the nuances of color. Yasper "drew" the flowers and leaves, emphasizing the shapes by outlining them with a slightly darker shade. Finally, when the colored ink had dried, he used a very fine brush to add the pistils of the flowers. He worked with concentration throughout the session. He sat hunched over his work, and as time passed, he raised his shoulders more and more.

During the brief reflection, the therapist asked how Yasper had worked today. He sighed deeply and indicated that it was quite exhausting. The therapist compared his work with the example and asked what it was like to continue with the example. Yasper said that he actually wanted to "improve" the example by making the shapes clearer. When the therapist mentioned that this is quite difficult with such fluid material, he indicated that he was working very intensely. When the therapist asked what it was like to do that, he first said, "Well, okay." The therapist stated that she observed some tension in his body and he recognized that. He didn't like it when the colored ink just didn't stay tight in the form. When the therapist asked if he recognized this feeling in the session, he said no, he just wanted to do it as well as possible.

After this session, the therapist added the observations to the notes made after the first observation session. Also, based on these three sessions, the therapist already had a first impression of patterns of material interaction, material experience, and the art product (see Table 4.1). Among other things, the therapist noticed that Yasper needed outside guidance and had a strong tendency to control the material. She also noticed that he set the bar very high for himself and that he was extremely tense while working and did not seem to recognize that. She wondered if Yasper would be able to let go of control a bit, how he would experience this, and if he himself felt any difference in feelings from the previous sessions. This was taken into account in the instruction for the next session.

4.5   Observations during session 4: observation session 3

The fourth session was again a group assignment, with each client working on the same assignment. Since control seemed to be an issue for Yasper as well as for several clients in this group, the therapist had chosen watercolors with structured and simple instructions. Each client was given a board with a 30 × 50 cm/ 12 × 20 inches sheet of watercolor paper taped to it. The task was to make color transitions. First, the therapist briefly explained the material: the less paint on the brush and the more mixed with water, the lighter the color. The therapist pointed out that they could choose the direction of the paper. The therapist also asked the clients to choose two colors of watercolor that they liked. Some clients had

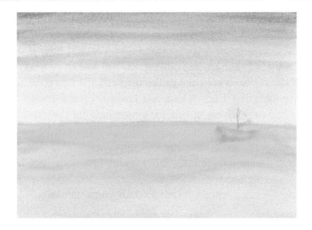

Image 4.3 Art product in observation session 3.

difficulty making a choice, including Yasper. The therapist suggested choosing colors that are close together, such as red and yellow, dark blue and light blue, yellow and green. Yasper chose dark blue and light blue (see Image 4.3).

The therapist then asked Yasper to wet the entire sheet of paper with a sponge and indicated that he could work standing up. Yasper said he thought this was a little crazy. He then continued to gently wipe the sponge across the paper until the therapist said it was sufficiently wet.

The therapist then asked Yasper to take the brush and start at the top of the paper with a color. The idea was to make a color transition from dark to light to about the middle of the paper. The therapist suggested moving the brush horizontally. Yasper started with dark blue. He made short, slow horizontal movements. The therapist suggested making the movements longer, moving the brush from the far left to the far right and back again, working downward. Yasper then made longer horizontal movements and more from a loose wrist. When he reached the middle of the paper, he indicated that there was not much difference between the top and the bottom. The therapist reminded him of the "the more color, the darker" explanation. Yasper continued to stand and applied more paint to the top and again worked toward the middle. He looked relaxed. The therapist then asked him to do the same again with the other color, starting from the center of the paper. Yasper continued to make long horizontal movements. Gradually, he said it was beginning to look like a sea and made slightly more wavy movements. He also "drew" a boat with it, but it flowed out. Yasper was clearly balking, tension was rising. Yasper began to tidy up.

During the reflection, the therapist asks how everyone experienced the material that day. Yasper indicated that he actually thought it was "cool" at first, "… until that little boat…" The therapist asked further: "How did you get started?" The tension seemed to ease a bit as Yasper indicated that he enjoyed working with the task and that he worked calmly. The therapist mentioned, "Although the material is a bit like the colored ink, it's also hard to control, especially since you were working on a wet surface..." "Yes, but now it didn't have to stay within the lines," said Yasper, adding, "It just had to be a color transition." The therapist asked, "So what's the difference with the flower branch?" "That it doesn't have to look like that." "Does that lower the bar for you?" the therapist asked. Yasper had to think about this for a moment, but then said, "Yes, I think so...in a way it does." The therapist said, "On the way over, I heard you say that you thought it looked like a seascape." "Right, yes." "And then I noticed that you also made different movements, more undulating, look here [pointing to in the picture]... you started with short movements, then longer movements, and here undulating." Yasper replied, "That actually came naturally." "And how was that?" "Well, that came naturally." The therapist said, "I had the impression that you were more relaxed than in the previous sessions...?" "Yes, until that little boat..." "Then what happened?" "Yes, because it became a seascape, I thought it would be nice to have a little boat in it, but that completely flowed out." The therapist agreed, "Yes, the paper wasn't dry yet." Yasper replied, "Yeah, not so cool!" to which the therapist said, "No, I get it, you tried to do something that didn't work because the surface was still wet." "Yes... I tried to fix it anyway, but it just made it worse. Then I just stopped." Fellow client M. said she liked the little boat: "It fits the image that it is not so tightly drawn, and you still recognize that it is a boat." Yasper didn't see it that way.

After this session, the therapist filled in the ArTA observation form with the context of the session, the material interaction, the material experience, and the reflection of this second session. And, again, determined the structure and variation of the art product based on the formal elements of movement, dynamic, contour, repetition, mixture of color, and color saturation (see Table 4.1).

This completed Step 1, Observing. The therapist decided, prior to the overall reflection with Yasper, to first analyze the patterns of Yasper's material interaction material experience and the structure and variation of his art product (Step 2, Analyzing). She noted these on the ArTA observation form, knowing that she could make any additions based on the joint reflection. This also allowed her to begin to interpret these patterns in terms of balance and adaptability. She did not write these on the ArTA observation form yet because she wanted to reflect with Yasper first.

4.6 Findings during the overall reflection

For overall reflection, the therapist had hung the three art products side by side. They looked at them together. The therapist asked how they worked. "The first one was the worst," said Yasper. When the therapist asked why, he said he didn't like the fact that the colors of the colored ink flowed together so easily. The therapist pointed out that, in the example of the blossom branch, the blossoms in particular were created on the basis of flow and chance and that this characterizes the image very much. She asked why he chose that particular example. Yasper explained that the image made him think of Japan: "For me, there's something about Japan." The therapist asked if it was not his intention to reproduce the example exactly. Yasper indicated that this was the intention indeed, but that somehow it seemed better to him if the colors did not touch. The therapist looked at him questioningly and he replied, "Yes, otherwise I can't control how it turns out." And when the therapist asked if that would be bad, he said, "I didn't mind if it was different from the example, but I wanted to control it." The therapist asked how that worked out. "Well…it didn't…" And what it was like then? "Not so relaxed…" The therapist asked why he was so eager to finish the flower branch. "When I start something, I want to finish it." Yasper explained. "Even if it makes you uncomfortable?" the therapist asked. Surprise appeared on Yasper's face. The therapist explained, "The tension increased while you were working on the flower branch, but you continued. Didn't it occur to you to change your plan?" Yasper understood what the therapist meant, but said that he only saw it now in retrospect; it did not occur to him while he was working.

The therapist mentioned that in the second picture he also seemed to have a clear plan by first putting a dot of color on all the surfaces. Yasper agreed and said that he thought it was very important to have a plan. "Yet I saw less tension than in the blossom branch," the therapist stated. "True… but that was because of the material." Yasper replied. The therapist continued: "Then what is it about the material?" "Acrylic was easier for me to control." "And you liked that?" "Yes, I did, yes." The therapist wondered aloud if the lower tension was just because the material was more controllable and made the comparison with the first and last picture: "Here you also worked with a fluid material. But here I saw less tension…" Yasper reflected: "Well, I liked the assignment…" "How did you work here? And what was different from the flower branch?" asked the therapist. "Yes, here we had to make a color transition and I let the color flow," said Yasper. "Yes, indeed," the therapist agreed, adding: "Here [pointing to the flower branch] you tried to control the material, which wasn't really possible, fluid material is hard to control. And here you just let the material do its thing". Yasper nodded… "Except here [pointing to the boat]." "What happened here?" the therapist asked. Yasper replied, "Yeah, that just failed and ruined the whole work…. I thought it was so funny what M. said… I've been thinking about that too; why can't I see it that way?"

The therapist replied, "The way I see it, you want to do very well. So well that sometimes you make it very difficult, even impossible for yourself. Colored ink [pointing to the blossom branch] just cannot be controlled, and neither can painting a boat in watercolor on a wet surface. [Yasper chuckled a little]. Then the tension rises. And I get the impression that you're not really thinking about it. You just keep going, and you don't see any other way." Yasper nodded. The therapist gave him some space and then asked if he recognized this in other situations. "Totally. Then I get all twisted up and can't see a way out." "And then?" "Then I get angry, but I don't know what else to do. Then I get sad." The therapist asked what Yasper himself would like to change. He didn't really know, but "Something has to change."

Based on this shared reflection, the therapist was able to complete the ArTA observation form. She completed Step 3, Interpreting, and formulated the ArTA assessment (Step 4, Formulating). She attempted to support her conclusions with observations of patterns in Yasper's material interaction, material experience, structure, and variation of his art products. She also included the findings from the reflection with Yasper, including his own perspective and expressed needs (see Table 4.1). In formulating the ArTA assessment, she was mindful to use a language that would both reflect her observations of Yasper and the specifics of art therapy, and be understandable to her colleagues who were also involved in Yasper's treatment. After discussion among the treatment team, it was decided that Yasper would continue to receive art therapy. Based on the ArTA assessment, the therapist was able to formulate treatment goals and determine how the treatment would be structured and which art therapy interventions would be used. Before starting treatment, she discussed this approach with Yasper. He agreed with the suggested approach and found it both exciting and hopeful to begin at the same time.

Table 4.1 Completed ArTA observation form of Yasper

ArTA Observation Form			
GENERAL INFORMATION			
Name: Yasper **Age:** 37 years **Reason for application therapy program:** depressive symptoms **Date:**			
CONTEXT OF THE SESSION			
	Sessions 1 and 3	Session 2	Session 4
Material, technique, and tools used What material, technique, and tools were used? Was it chosen by the client or provided by the therapist? What was the size of the paper?	Colored ink on watercolor paper measuring 32 × 40 cm (12 × 16 inches). Material was chosen based on the example chosen by the client. There was a wide range of art material to choose from, ranging from solid to fluid.	Acrylic paint with brushes on thick 30 × 50 cm (14 × 20 inches) drawing paper on which the therapist has taped a 25 × 50 cm (10 × 20 inches) frame. Materials, tools, and acrylic paint were provided by the therapist.	Materials and technique provided by the therapist: watercolor, wet-in-wet technique with brushes on 30 × 50 cm (14 × 20 inches), watercolor paper taped to a board.
Instruction How much direction did the client need to start art-making?	No instruction, client chooses an example from a book. Therapist gives no instruction but recommends the use of colored ink.	Group assignment: creating a division into planes based on initials on paper onto which a frame is added with crepe tape. The planes were worked in with acrylic paint.	Group assignment: making color transitions by applying watercolor from dark to light with a brush.

(Continued)

Table 4.1 (Continued)

MATERIAL INTERACTION			
	Sessions 1 and 3	**Session 2**	**Session 4**
Movement Especially, the *size* of movements (small to large), *direction* of movement (outward or inward-facing), and *type* of movement (curved or straight; vertical, horizontal, or diagonal).	Short, sketchy, diagonal movements to reproduce the branch as accurately as possible.	Initials with pencil appropriately set up within the frame. Adds 1 curved line itself. Short movements when filling in with acrylic paint, in the direction of the plane.	Short and long, straight and wavy, horizontal movements (in agreement with instruction).
Pressure The degree of *physical pressure* (light to heavy) and the degree of *focus* (alert and attentive to unfocused).	No standouts regarding physical pressure (not an issue with colored ink). Works with great attention.	With pencil first little strength, then traced firmly with ruler. With acrylic paint no standouts. Works attentively, focused, and precisely.	No standouts. Works with attention.
Grip The manner in which the material is *held* (loose with loose wrists to strong with wrist and/or fingers).	Handles the brush from the wrist, holding it firmly.	Holds the brush firmly.	First from fixed, later with looser wrist.
Tempo The *speed* at which the client works (fast or slow).	Slow.	Quietly, slowly. When filling in the areas a little faster.	Slow.
Rhythm The *continuity* of actions in time (repetitious, continuous, or variable, interrupted).	He worked continuously, took no distance, continuously focused on the work. Lots of repetition (first the shape, then the outline, then the details).	He worked continuously; his actions were repetitive; he filled in the planes in the same way.	Lots of repetition (following instruction) and some variety in lines.

(Continued)

Table 4.1 (Continued)

	Sessions 1 and 3	Session 2	Session 4
Organization The degree to which the client organizes their art-making process (planned, thoughtful or chaotic, impulsive) and activity (passive, casual, or actively initiating).	Thoughtful and planned; he stopped the movement before a recess in the branch. Tried to imitate the example as best he could and very precisely. He worked in an organized order but deviated from the example; he wanted to make it better.	Organized and planned: first marking the areas with color, then the outline/ contour and, then working in. Color choice seemed to be coincidental.	Allowed himself to be structured by the steps in the assignment.
Physical contact The extent to which fingers/ hands make contact with the material (non-fingertip to whole hand) and the manner (smearing, rubbing, etc.)	No standouts.	No standouts.	No standouts.
Space *How much* space the actions require in relation to the paper/canvas of the art product and the amount of material used.	No standouts. Seemed to be somewhat short of space at the top.	Used the entire framework (inherent in instruction).	Used the entire paper but stopped at the edges (following instruction).
Lining The *degree* of line use (a lot or little) and *type* of line use (sketchy/ interrupted or lined/flowing).	Many lines; he worked sketching with the brush and colored ink. Many outlines especially in the blossoms.	With acrylic paint first outline: lining.	Created many lines, flowing into each other through the wet-on-wet technique.
Mixing colors The *degree* of mixing during art making (none, colors are used separately or a lot).	He worked with dilution to recreate light and dark as closely as possible according to the example. There was no mixing of color in the thinner branches and blossoms.	No color mixing: colors were used directly from the jar.	Relatively large amount of mixing of color by dilution (following instruction).

(Continued)

Table 4.1 (Continued)

	Sessions 1 and 3	Session 2	Session 4
Shaping Removing and/or adding material (removing or adding).	No standouts.	No standouts.	Added an extra layer to darken the color.
Dialogue The degree of exploration: searching, experimenting, and playing with the properties and possibilities of the material (versus wanting to control it).	He tried to control/ direct the colored ink. He used it like a pencil: he "drew" with it. The color nuances present were functional (to make it look like the example) and controlled.	No dialogue, wanted to control the material. He tried the thicker brush for filling in areas but did not try the different properties of the material.	Appropriate to the assignment. "Drawing" the little boat was outside the instruction but showed little dialogue; would like to control it.
Material Interaction Style *Combination* of the categories (positioning on continuum of rational to affective).	The combination of working by example, wanting to make it even better than the example, the structured manner in which he worked, the attention and precision with which he worked, and the lack of dialogue with the material points to a more rational material interaction style.	Seemed to want to control the material through the rigid lines, repetition in acting, failure to dialogue with the material. Combined with the thoughtfulness in his actions and slow pace, this resembles a more rational material interaction style.	Following the instructions, the idea of a seascape arose to which he added an additional element. He worked slowly. Followed the structure of the assignment in which he showed more dialogue with the material, yet still a more rational style of material interaction.

PATTERN OF MATERIAL INTERACTION
Overall pattern (consistency across sessions) positioning on continuum of rational to affective.

Copy this section to "Overview of all patterns" below.

Y. demonstrated a rational pattern of material interaction in which the need for structure and control became evident. He worked thoughtfully, planned, and organized. He liked to have an outside structure (example/assignment) and he did not deviate from his plan. He wanted to perfect the example. There was little room for dialogue with the material from within himself: there was no exploration, but the material was strongly controlled. In the context of an assignment, he could engage in a little more dialogue with the material.

(Continued)

Table 4.1 (Continued)

MATERIAL EXPERIENCE			
	Sessions 1 and 3	**Session 2**	**Session 4**
The way in which the client experiences the art material and the extent to which the client can recognize, allow, adequately express, and regulate this feeling (body posture, facial expressions, verbal expression, etc.) Does this involve a difference between positive and negative emotions? Any preferences of the client; does the client prefer to choose solid materials that can be easily controlled or does the client prefer to work with more fluid materials?	Y. chose material that fitted best to recreate the example. Despite the fact that this was a fluid material, he made little use of this characteristic and tried to strongly control it. Afterward, he mentioned the concentration and energy this required of him, and the fatigue and tension while working, Also, that he did not notice this so much in the moment. The focus was on wanting to do well and finish. So he ignored these sensations and carried on.	Y. could indicate that acrylic paint was easier to control than colored ink and mentioned that he liked it. He also indicated that he liked being given an assignment. That gave him clarity.	Y. recognized that he has worked more relaxed but put a strong focus on the moment he felt something did not work out. He considered that a failure.

PATTERN OF MATERIAL EXPERIENCE
Overall pattern (consistency across sessions) in relation to the context of the
session (difference in material (fluid-solid), technique, size, instruction).

Are feelings recognized, allowed, and expressed? What is in the foreground?

Copy this section to "Overview of all patterns" below.

Y. had difficulty recognizing the tension involved in controlling fluid material. His focus
was so much on the creation of a (beautiful) end result that he may have ignored it.
Controlling the material created a paradox: instead of giving him a sense of direction
and control, it actually led to tension. He did not recognize it during the art-making,
and it therefore lingered somewhat in feelings of fatigue, tension, and sadness.

He enjoyed working within a provided structure (assignment) and became more aware
of the difference between materials. Negative feelings of fatigue, tension, failure, and
sadness predominate.

(Continued)

Table 4.1 (Continued)

	Sessions 1 and 3 Art Product 1	Session 2 Art Product 2	Session 4 Art Product 3
Movement The *degree of* movement (none to a lot). Movement becomes visible in the brushstroke/ line-work.	Some movement due to the diagonal of the branch and the brush stroke. Otherwise little to no movement.	Very little movement.	Some degree of movement in line with instruction, especially in the bottom of the image.
Dynamic The *tension* in the image (tectonic to atectonic) varying from calm and static to energetic, turbulent, and powerful. It reflects the *vitality* of movement.	The image looks static and somewhat convulsive. It stays within the framework of the support (tectonic). The movement stops and inhibits the dynamics.	There is no tension in the image. Static.	The image looks calm and tranquil.
Contour The *degree of* delineation of parts of the art product by outlining or tightly placed against each other (sharp delineation/linear to pictorial).	A lot of contour: shapes are tight and accentuated by lines. Within the branch less contour, somewhat pictorial.	Lots of contour: the color areas are set tightly together (somewhat in line with instruction).	Some contour due to center line (following instruction).
Repetition The *degree* to which one or more elements are repeated in a pattern (symmetry/rhythm or no repetition/ overall).	Some repetition through the linework/brush stroke.	No obvious repetition.	Lots of repetition.
Color mixture The *degree* to which colors are visibly mixed (none to a lot).	Some degree in the main branch (light to dark) of the same color shade. There was no color mixing in the thinner branches, leaves, and flowers.	No color mixing.	Quite a bit of color dilution as part of the instruction to make color transitions.

(Continued)

Table 4.1 (Continued)

	Sessions 1 and 3 Art Product 1	Session 2 Art Product 2	Session 4 Art Product 3
Color saturation The *degree* of saturation (transparent to impasto).	A relatively large amount of color saturation given the material.	Lots of color saturation.	No standouts.
Structure The degree of ordering of the art product based on the combination of formal elements (positioning on continuum high to low).	Relatively high structure.	High structure.	High structure.
Variation Degree of diversity of formal elements.	Some degree of variation in color saturation and color mixing, but appropriate to the example used.	No variation.	Some degree of variation in movement and color saturation. Addition of the boat.

PATTERN OF STRUCTURE
Overall pattern (consistency across art products): positioning on continuum of a lot of structure (rational) to no structure (affective).

Copy this section to "Overview of all patterns" below.

High structure: the art products have little to no movement, little dynamic (static, calm, and convulsive) and a lot of contour. This structure is reinforced in the first two art products by high color saturation and little color mixing. With clear instruction, he can loosen the structure somewhat because he likes to get it right.

PATTERN OF VARIATION
Overall pattern (consistency across art products): degree of diversity.

Copy this section to "Overview of all patterns" below.

Minimal to little variation. Some variation is recognizable in the color mixing and diversity in color saturation in the main branch of the first art product and in the movement and color saturation in the third art product.

(Continued)

Table 4.1 (Continued)

JOINT REFLECTION			
	Sessions 1 and 3	**Session 2**	**Session 4**
Reflection with the client on material interaction, material experience, choices, and preferences for materials and techniques, art product, and other. In the third session also reflection on client's wishes,	Recognized that the material is difficult to control and mentioned to have found this tiring, but nevertheless wanted to continue working. Recognized the tension the therapist mentioned. Afterward, he linked this to the	Indicated that he liked acrylic paint better because it was easier to control. Said he also liked working with an assignment. He also recognized the moment when his neighbor	Recognized the difference in tension between the beginning of the task and later when it as failure. Was surprised by the, more positive, perspective of his fellow client.
needs, preferences, expectations, and request for help.	moments when the material flowed. In the moment itself he did not think about it, he wanted to do it well.	started to mix color, which appealed to him, but he continued along the same path.	he wantewd to draw the boat. Focused strongly on that moment and labeled

REFLECTION OVERALL
Degree of reflectivity (translation to/relation to situations outside therapy)

Main reflections.

Other.

Copy this section to "Overview of all patterns" below.

Y. recognized the difference in materials and could indicate that he liked material that was easier to control. If he wanted to control material that was very difficult to control, tension arose. He realized that he was not aware of the tension in the moment. Only afterward did he feel tired, stressed, and sad. He desperately wanted to do well, but couldn't. This led to a sense of failure.

Together, Y. could also make the link to situations outside therapy. There, too, he fails to recognize tension in the moment and keeps going. He also recognized the great need to want to do things right and that he often wants to control something that cannot be controlled. He also named feelings of anger and despondency. Y. had no further concrete ideas or preferences for therapy but did indicate the need for change.

(Continued)

Table 4.1 (Continued)

OVERVIEW OF ALL PATTERNS			
Pattern of Material Interaction	**Pattern of Material** Experience	**Pattern of Structure and** Variation	**Reflection Overall**
Y. demonstrated a rational pattern of material interaction in which the need for structure and control became evident. He worked thoughtfully, planned, and organized. He liked to have an outside structure (example/ assignment) and he did not deviate from his plan. He wanted to perfect the example. There was little room for dialogue with the material from within himself: there was no exploration, but the material was strongly controlled. In the context of an assignment, he could engage in a little more dialogue with the material.	Y. had difficulty recognizing the tension involved in controlling fluid material. His focus was so much on the creation of a (beautiful) end result that he may have ignored it. Controlling the material created a paradox: instead of giving him a sense of direction and control, it actually led to tension. He did not recognize it during the art-making, and it therefore lingered somewhat in feelings of fatigue, tension, and sadness. He enjoyed working within a provided structure (assignment) and became more aware of the difference between materials. Negative feelings of fatigue, tension, failure, and sadness predominate.	High structure: the art products have little to no movement, little dynamic (static, calm, and convulsive), and a lot of contour. This structure is reinforced in the first two art products by high color saturation and little color mixing. With clear instruction, he can loosen the structure somewhat because he likes to get it right. Minimal to little variation. Some variation is recognizable in the color mixing and diversity in color saturation in the main branch of the first art product and in the movement and color saturation in the third art product.	Y. recognized the difference in materials and could indicate that he liked material that was easier to control. If he wanted to control material that was very difficult to control, tension arose. He realized that he was not aware of the tension in the moment. Only afterward did he feel tired, stressed, and sad. He desperately wanted to do well but couldn't. This led to a sense of failure. Together, Y. could also make the link to situations outside therapy. There, too, he fails to recognize tension in the moment and keeps going. He also recognized the great need to want to do things right and that he often wants to control something that cannot be controlled. He also named feelings of anger and despondency. Y. had no further concrete ideas or preferences for therapy but did indicate the need for change.

(Continued)

Table 4.1 (Continued)

ArTA ASSESSMENT
Yasper shows a clear rational pattern of material interaction and, thus, an imbalance toward thinking: he approaches situations art therapy strongly "from the head." From a strong need to want to do things right, he works in a thoughtful, planned, and organized way, focusing strongly on the result and preferably with a benchmark outside himself. He ignores his own feelings: has difficulty recognizing them in the moment. He has a clear need for a sense of control and direction, even in situations that cannot be controlled. Apart from the fact that he is barely in touch with his own feelings, he is then also minimally indialogue with the art material, as a result of which he does not feel wherehis limit lies.
This leads to tension, fatigue, despondency, and anger. In a structured safe situation, he can engage in a little more dialogue with the material.
Yasper demonstrates limited **adaptability**. Because of the strong tendency to approach things from the head and the difficulty in recognizing and admitting feelings, it is difficult for Yasper to adapt his actions **flexibly** to a variety of situations. He continues on his chosen path, even when it is not pleasant.
He prefers to work with a benchmark outside himself and wants to do very well, so he makes few choices of his own. In the moment, he pays little attention to his feelings as a signal function, which prevents him from adjusting his choices and actions in the moment. This demonstrates limited **self-management**.
He is open to suggestions from the therapist and tries them out, but in doing so, he hardly engages in dialogue with the art material. He strongly emphasizes what is not going well and finds it difficult to look at it from a different perspective. This limits his **openness**.
He does not seem to allow himself any space to explore new possibilities and to explore and to see situations from different perspectives. He prefers not to take risks and not to deviate from his chosen path. In a structured situation, he succeeds somewhat. As a result, his **creativity** is limited.
Yasper shows a fair degree of reflection. He recognizes what the therapist mentions and can also make the link with situations outside the therapy.
He recognizes that he mostly conforms to benchmarks outside of himself, not dwelling on feelings this evokes in him. He also recognizes his need for control, even things that may not be controllable. And that this leads to feelings of being stuck, fatigue, tension, anger, and despondency. He does not know how to deal with this. Regarding his own perspective, Yasper has no explicit expectation, preference, or idea for follow-up treatment. He feels a great need for change but does not know how. He does indicate that he would like to learn to see things from a different, more positive perspective.

(Continued)

Table 4.1 (Continued)

Art therapy is **indicated** to restore balance and increase adaptability.

- Yasper could benefit from gaining (steady) affective experience through art therapy to become less dependent on cognitive control and more in touch with his own feelings. Experiencing that letting go of control is not frightening will help him to use feeling more as a signaling function. This will teach him to listen to himself rather than to a standard outside of himself. If he can make conscious deliberations from a calmer place, he will gain more control over his own decisions and actions (self-management), which will allow him to be more flexible with his environment.

- In a structured environment, Yasper will be able to benefit from the opportunity that art-making provides to look at situations from different perspectives. By pausing in a safe context and daring to allow for feelings and bodily reactions, working with different materials, including those that are less controllable, contributes to adaptive capacity. Discovering the different possibilities of art materials provides space for exploration and relaxation. Experiencing that trying something new does not immediately lead to disaster gives room to look at situations from multiple perspectives. Yasper himself indicates a need for more rest and relaxation and, therefore, seems motivated for treatment.

Goals that would be appropriate here are:

- Restoring balance between thinking and feeling:

  o Gaining positive affective experiences in a structured setting.
  o Recognizing and admitting (negative) feelings

- Increase adaptive capacity:

  o Being able to use feelings as signals to adjust behavior, thus increasing flexibility.
  o Not seeing "mistakes" as failures but looking at situations from different perspectives and seeing possibilities and, thus, increasing openness and creativity.
  o Learning to make more considered choices and, thus, increasing self-management.

Art therapy is offered with a frequency of 2 × one and a half hours per week, of which one is group therapy and one is individual therapy, for a period of 6 weeks. An extension of 6 weeks is possible.

Epilogue

I have found that translating scientific findings into a practical method is a creative process in itself. So is writing a book about it! It had to be delineated. And as a researcher, I cannot help but be critical of some aspects. I would like to take you through some of these considerations.

The research findings are based on a large number of art therapists with different theoretical background and perspectives and an even larger number of adult clients with different mental health issues. Therefore, ArTA transcends different art therapy approaches and is widely applicable with adults. One question I am often asked is whether ArTA can be used with children. It is not unreasonable to wonder to what extent these findings can be transferred to another (age) group, and the conceptual framework of ArTA is, indeed, generic. However, I am also a strong advocate of critical thinking. By that I mean that we must also be cautious about translating research findings from one group of clients to clients of different ages and with different needs.

In the case of children, development plays an important role. I am referring, in particular, to the development of drawing and art-making, which occurs in children in fixed stages. In my opinion, this development affects the observation of material interaction, material experience, and the art product. This requires further research.

Similar questions can be asked when using ArTA with older clients, where degenerative processes may be involved, or with clients with psychotic problems. After all, the group of clients in the ArTA study were all between the ages of 18 and 68, and clients with psychotic problems were excluded from participation. This means that we don't know how these factors affect observation and assessment. This shows that research leads to knowledge, but it also leads to new questions. Worthy of further research.

I am also sometimes asked if ArTA can be used more broadly than just at the beginning or during monitoring of art therapy. The insight into the (im)balance between thinking and feeling and the adaptability is also relevant for people who do not directly need help within the mental health care system, but who still want to get better. I am thinking of people who want to get the best out of themselves or learn to cope better with stress and other challenges that life brings. For example, in learning and work situations.

I think ArTA can also play a role in the prevention of disease. By detecting possible imbalances early and keeping an eye on adaptability, you can prevent someone from becoming so unbalanced that they are temporarily unable to work or study.

I also think that ArTA can be used as a complement to regular (verbal) forms of HR assessment, for example in the context of recruitment and selection and talent development.

One of my main motivations for conducting this research was to contribute to the art therapy body of knowledge. If this book finds its way into education and practice, I will have come full circle. Experience shows that it is through education that knowledge really comes to life. That is why I offer various ArTA (continuing education) programs. Check out my website "Where Art meets Health": www.ingridpenzes.com.

Ingrid Pénzes

Appendix 1

Extended definitions of formal elements of art products on a five-point scale

The tables below provide the detailed descriptions of the formal elements on a five-point scale, as used in the ArTA survey. These may be helpful if you are new to observing formal elements, or if you are unsure about the formal elements in a product.

MOVEMENT The amount and direction of movement in the image, ranging from little to a large amount. Movement is evident in the brushstroke/linework.	
1 = no	There is **no** movement in the art product. The art product looks completely static.
2 = low	There is little movement in the art product. There are few and/or small movements recognizable in the brushstroke/line work, in mostly the same direction, without overlap. The image looks calm and stable, but **not entirely static**.
3 = average	There is **average** movement in the art product. The art product does not look entirely static, but neither does it look entirely moving.
4 = high	There is **a lot** of movement in the art product. The art product looks moving.
5 = very high	There is a lot of movement in the art product. There are a lot of and/or large movements in different directions that can be recognized in the brush stroke/line work. Possibly there is overlap. The art product looks **very moving**.

DYNAMIC

The tension in the image, ranging from little to a large amount. It reflects the vitality of the movement. This tension arises because the image appears to step outside its frame (frame de-tectonic*).

* The elements in the image seem to deny the frame (edges of the paper); they splash off the paper, as it were. This is in contrast to frame-affirming, where the elements clearly remain within the frame.

1 = no	There is **no tension at all** in the art product. The art product shows calmness, a peaceful coexistence between the image itself and the space around it, without prying determined by frame. All elements of the art product remain entirely within the frame. The dynamic is characterized by complete **tranquility**.
2 = low	There is **little tension** in the art product. The art product exhibits calmness but shows a denial of the frame at certain portions of the image. A small number of lines or planes could seemingly continue beyond the frame. For the most part, the dynamics are **quiet and calm**.
3 = average	There is **average** tension in the art product. The art product is not clearly characterized by total tranquility or by total tension. The art product is not frame-denying, but neither is it frame-affirming. Elements of the art product as a whole might extend beyond the frame but do not produce tension between the overall image and the frame. The dynamic is **lively and harmonious**.
4 = high	There is **a lot** of tension in the art product. The art product as a whole is largely frame-denying, but in a small number of parts, the lines and planes within the frame or do not deliver ultimate tension. The dynamic is **energetic**.
5 = very high	The overall art product is characterized by **a great deal** of tension between image and frame; the art product is completely and utterly frame-denying. The image seems to be restrained with friction by the frame. The dynamic is **restless and turbulent**.

CONTOUR
The degree of delineation of parts of the art product by outlining or tightly placing shapes against each other, ranging from little to a large amount.

1 = no	There is **no** contour in the art product. The art product as a whole makes a pictorial, diffuse, shrouded, vague, and woolly impression.
2 = low	There is **little** contour in the art product. This means that some surfaces can be recognized, but the delineation is not sharp (think of a sketchy edge), rather sketchy, friable, or tarnished. Most of the art product shows no contour.
3 = average	Lines or planes may be present, without a clear contour, but they are also not completely without contour. This means that the art product consists of elements that are all clearly recognizable, but whose demarcation is not sharp. **Or**: in the art product, an equal part (half) is woolly (without contour), and an equal part is sharply delineated (clear contour).
4 = high	There is **a lot** of contour. This means that in the art product there are largely clearly delineated elements, but not entirely sharply delineated (contour lines, for example, do not run all the way through, the demarcation between color areas is not ultimately sharp).
5 = very high	**Throughout** the whole image, there are very obvious contours; contour lines are clearly visible and outline completely the shape(s) and are tight and flowing. **Or**: areas of color are tightly set against each other. Color contrasts are overtly present. The obvious contours are very defining to the image.

REPETITION
The degree to which one or more elements are repeated in a pattern, ranging from few to many.

1 = no	**No** rhythm can be recognized in the art product. The art product has no repetition of line, shape, color, or structure.
2 = low	The art product has **little** rhythm. This means that in the art product an element is repeated exactly, but to a limited extent, so that one cannot speak of a rhythmic pattern.
3 = average	The art product is **moderately** rhythmic. This means that the overall art product has some rhythmic elements through which some repetition can be recognized, but there is no rhythmic pattern in the art product.
4 = high	The art product has **a lot** of rhythm. The art product contains a clear rhythmic pattern, but it is not fully implemented in the overall art product.
5 = very high	The art product has **a lot** of repetition. The art product contains one or more distinct rhythmic patterns. These patterns involve all elements of the art product (color, shape, line, structure). They characterize the art product **as a whole**.

MIXTURE OF COLOR
The degree to which colors are visibly mixed, ranging from none to a large
amount.

1 = no	There is **no** color mixing in the art product. Colors in the art product are separate from each other.
2 = low	There is **hardly** any color mixing. This means that the colors in the art product are largely unmixed, only a few colors are minimally mixed.
3 = average	There is **average** color mixing in the art product. This means that there are an equal number of colors not mixed as colors that are mixed. **Or**: that many colors are mixed but minimal in color mixing.
4 = high	There is **a lot** of color mixing. This means that in the art product most of the colors are mixed.
5 = very high	There is a lot of color mixing. The art product consists of **almost only** mixed colors.

COLOR SATURATION	
The degree of saturation, ranging from little to a large amount.	
1 = no	There is **no** color saturation at all. All the colors in the art product are unsaturated; there is a lot of the paper still visible.
2 = low	There is **little** color saturation. This means that only some of the colors in the pictorial product are fully saturated. **Or**: All colors in the art product are minimally saturated, but not completely unsaturated as in 1.
3 = average	There is **average** color saturation. This means that: The colors in the art product are not fully saturated but also not fully unsaturated. There is an equal portion of the paper visible through the color. **Or**: There is an equal distribution of colors in the art product applied transparently or saturated.
4 = high	There is **a lot** of color saturation. This means that: Most of the colors in the art product are fully saturated, except for a few colors. **Or**: That all the colors in the art product are almost fully saturated, but some of the paper is still visible.
5 = very high	**All** colors in the image are **fully** saturated.

Appendix 2

ArTA observation form

ArTA OBSERVATION FORM			
GENERAL INFORMATION			
Name: **Age:** **Reason for application therapy program**: **Date:**			
CONTEXT OF THE SESSION			
	Session 1	**Session 2**	**Session 3**
Material, technique and tools used What material, technique, and tools were used? Was it chosen by the client or provided by the therapist? What was the size of the paper?			
Instruction How much direction did the client need to start art-making?			
MATERIAL INTERACTION			
Movement Especially the *size* of movements (small to large), *direction* of movement (outward or inward-facing), and *type* of movement (curved or straight, vertical or horizontal, or diagonal).			
Pressure The degree of *physical pressure* (light to heavy) and the degree of *focus* (alert and attentive to unfocused).			

	Session 1	Session 2	Session 3
Grip The manner in which the material is *held* (loose with loose wrists to strong with wrist and/or fingers).			
Tempo The *speed* at which the client works (fast or slow).			
Rhythm The *continuity* of actions in time (repetitious, continuous or variable, interrupted).			
Organization The degree to which the client organizes their art-making process (planned, thoughtful to chaotic, impulsive) and activity (passive, casual, or actively initiating).			
Physical contact The extent to which fingers/ hands make contact with the material (none or fingertip to whole hand) and the manner (smearing, rubbing, etc.)			
Space *How much* space the actions require in relation to the paper/canvas of the art product and the amount of material used.			
Lining The *degree* of line use (a lot or little) and *type* of line use (sketchy/interrupted or lined/ flowing).			

	Session 1	Session 2	Session 3
Mixing colors The *degree* of mixing during art making (none, colors are used separately or a lot).			
Shaping Removing and/or adding material (removing or adding).			
Dialogue The degree of exploration: searching, experimenting, and playing with the properties and possibilities of the material (versus wanting to control it).			
Material Interaction Style *Combination* of the categories (positioning on continuum of rational to affective).			

PATTERN OF MATERIAL INTERACTION

Overall pattern (consistency across sessions) positioning on continuum of rational to affective.

Copy this section to "Overview of all patterns" below.

MATERIAL EXPERIENCE

	Session 1	Session 2	Session 3
The way in which the client experiences the art material and the extent to which the client can recognize, allow, adequately express, and regulate this feeling (body posture, facial expressions, verbal expression, etc.) Does this involve a difference between positive and negative emotions? Any preferences of the client; does the client prefer to choose solid materials that can be easily controlled or does the client prefer to work with more fluid materials?			

PATTERN OF MATERIAL EXPERIENCE

Overall pattern (consistency across sessions) in relation to the context of the session (difference in material (fluid-solid), technique, size, instruction).

Are feelings recognized, allowed, and expressed? What is in the foreground?

Copy this section to "Overview of all patterns" below.

ART PRODUCT			
	Art Product 1	Art Product 2	Art Product 3
Movement The *degree* of movement (none to a lot). Movement becomes visible in the brushstroke/ line-work.			
Dynamic The *tension* in the image (tectonic to atectonic) varying from calm, calm, and static to energetic, turbulent, and powerful. It reflects the *vitality* of movement.			
Contour The *degree* of delineation of parts of the art product by outlining or tightly placed against each other (sharp delineation/ linear to pictorial).			
Repetition The *degree* to which one or more elements are repeated in a pattern (symmetry/ rhythm to no repetition/ overall).			
Color mixture The *degree* to which colors are visibly mixed (none to a lot).			

	Art Product 1	Art Product 2	Art Product 3
Color saturation The *degree* of saturation (transparent to impasto).			
Structure The degree of ordering of the art product based on the combination of formal elements (positioning on continuum high to low).			
Variation Degree of diversity of formal elements.			

PATTERN OF STRUCTURE

Overall pattern (consistency across art products): positioning on continuum of a lot of structure (rational) to no structure (affective).

Copy this section to "Overview of all patterns" below.

PATTERN OF VARIATION

Overall pattern (consistency across art products): degree of diversity.

Copy this section to "Overview of all patterns" below.

JOINT REFLECTION			
	Session 1	**Session 2**	**Session 3**
Reflection with the client on material interaction, material experience, choices and preferences for materials and techniques, art product, and other. In the 3rd session also reflection on client's wishes, needs, preferences, expectations, and request for help.			

REFLECTION OVERALL
Degree of reflectivity (translation to/relation to situations outside therapy)
Main reflections.
Other.

Copy this section to "Overview of all patterns" below.

OVERVIEW OF ALL PATTERNS

Pattern of Material Interaction	Pattern of Material Experience	Pattern of Structure and Variation	Overall Reflection

ArTA ASSESSMENT

Direction and degree of balance/imbalance: what patterns become apparent (direction of thinking to feeling) and how fixed are they.

Degree of adaptability in general:
Specified by:
Openness:
Flexibility:
Self-management:
Creativity:

Reflective capacity and perspective for further treatment:

Indication for further treatment, including the preferences, wishes, expectations, and needs of the client:

Treatment goals:

Prognosis:

Index

Note: **Bold** page numbers refer to tables and *italic* page numbers refer to figures.

adaptability: definition 12, *13*; from a neuroscientific perspective 15–22; in indication 69–71; relationship with balance *14*; in relation to material interaction and material experience *61*; in relation to the art product 45, 53; in step 3: Interpreting 84; in step 4: Formulating 86, 87
affective experience **19**, 20
affective pattern of material interaction 60, 85
affective style of material interaction 31, 43, 58, 85
amygdala 16
analogies 17
analogous processes 18
analogue process model 18
analytical art therapy 34, **35**, 37
analyzing *see* step 2: Analyzing
approaches to art therapy 29, 34, **35–36**, 37–38
approaches to mental health *see* mental health
art as therapy 1, **36**, 38
art form 3, 15
art in therapy 34, **35**, 37
art materials 1, 3, 4, 6, *7*, 31, 34, 51
art product 2, 3, 6, 15; *see also* formal elements; structure of the art product; variation
art psychotherapy 34, **35**, 37
art therapy 1–2
art therapy triangle 2–4
ArTA observation form 77–78, **117–120**
art-based approach 37

art-based assessments 37
art-based therapy **35**
art-making experience **19**
autonomic nervous system 16
autonomy 11

balance: definition 12, 32; from a neuroscientific perspective 15–22; in indication 69–71; relationship with adaptability 14; in relation to material interaction and material experience 61; in relation to the art product 45, 53; in step 3: Interpreting 84, 85; in step 4: Formulating 86, 87

categories of material interaction *see* material interaction
client 2
clinical reasoning 69
cognition 17, 18, 19, 22, 43, 71
cognitive control 12, 22, 30, 32; in indication 70; in step 3: Interpreting 85, 86
cognitive experience 18, **19**
combination of formal elements *see* formal elements
compassion 3, 17
complexity of instruction *see* instruction
context of art-making *4*–10, 51, 61
coping 13, 21, 31, 33
core-self 21
cortical processes 15–17, 22
cortisol 16
counter transference 34
creative art therapy **36**, 38

creativity 13–14, 33; in indication 70, 71; in step 3: Formulating 86; in step 4: Formulating 87

degree of instruction *see* instruction
Diagnostic and Statistical Manual of Mental Disorders (DSM) 10–11, 38
Diagnostic Assessment of Psychiatric Art (DAPA) **35**, 37
Diagnostic Drawing Series (DDS) **35**, 37
dysregulation 18, 20, 21

emotions 15, 17, 20, 31, 32, 59
evidence base 29, 30–34
experience 2, 3, 17, 18–20
experiential 13, 78
experiential acceptance 33
experiential qualities 18
Expressive Therapies Continuum (ETC) **36**, 38

feeling 12; from a neuroscientific perspective 17, 20 ,22; in indication 70; in reflection 67, 68; in relation to material interaction and material experience 43, 44, 59–61; in step 1: Observing 80; in step 2: Analyzing 83, 84; in step 3: Interpreting 85
flexibility: definition 13–14; in indication 70, 71; in step 4: Formulating 87; in step 3: Interpreting 86
Formal Elements Art Therapy Scale (FEATS) **35**, 37
formal elements: analyzing in the context of the session 51; in ArTA 39; in art-based approach 37; in creative art therapy approach 38; definition 45–47, **48–50**; in relation to movement 21; in relation to structure and variation *53–55*; in research 31–34
formulating *see* step 4: Formulating
four steps of ArTA *79*

health 11, 15
high-level instruction *see* instruction
hippocampus 16
history of art therapy observation and assessment 34, **35–36**, 37–38
House-Tree-Person Test (HTTP) **35**, 37
hypothalamic-pituitary-adrenal (HPA) axis 16
hypothalamus 16

iconological art analysis 46
identity 13
illness *see* mental health
imbalance 12; from neuroscientific perspective 17, 20; in indication 69–71; in movement 21; in relation to material interaction and art product 59–61; in step 4: Formulating 87; in step 3: Interpreting 84, 86
importance of experience *see* experience
importance of movement 21–22
indication 69–71
instruction 8, *9*, 61–64, **65**
integrating effect of art-making 22
integration 16, 17, 18, 19
interpreting *see* step 3: Interpreting
intervention 1, 20, 34, 60, 68; in indication 69, 70; in step 4: Formulating 87

limbic system 15–16
low-level instruction *see* instruction

material experience 30, 44–45; in indication 69–71; in relation to instruction 63–65; in relation to material interaction, art product and mental health 56, 59, 60, *61*; in relation to reflection 66; in step 1: Observing 79, 80; in step 2: Analyzing 82, 83; in step 3: Interpreting 84
material interaction 30, 31, 39, **40**, **41**, 42–44; in indication 69–71; in instruction 64–65; in reflection 66–67; in relation to material experience and art product 56, 58, *59*, 60, *61*; in relation to movement 21; in step 1: Observing 79–81; in step 2: Analyzing 83; in step 3: Interpreting 84–86
mental health 10–12; from neuroscientific perspective 15, 17, 18; in art therapy approaches 34, **35–36**, 38; in relation to material interaction, material experience and art product 45, 46, 53, *59*
mental resilience *see* resilience
methods of art therapy observation and assessment *see* approaches to art therapy
mixing panel 9, *10*
morphological art analysis 46

movement: as category of material interaction **40**, 41, 80; examples of movement in art products 54–55, 56–58; as formal element 47, **48**, 52, *53*, 81; *see also* importance of movement

neuroanalogous processes 14–18
neuroscientific approach to health *see* neuroanalogous processes
noncognitive level *see* subcortical processes
Nürtinger Rating Scale (NRS) **35**, 37

observing *see* step 1: observing
openness *13*–14, 32, 77; in indication 70, 71; in overall reflection 67, 84; in step 4: Formulating: 86, 87

parasympathetic nervous system *see* automatic nervous system
pathogenesis 10
patterns of material interaction 42–44
Person Picking an Apple from a Tree (PPAT) **35**, 37
positive health 11
(pre-) frontal cortex 16
Prognosis 43, 71
projective drawing tests 37
properties of art materials *see* art materials
psychological flexibility 11, 12
psychopathology 10

reflection 22, 66–68
regulation of emotions 16, 17
relationship between balance and adaptability *14*
relationship between material interaction, material experience, and art product 57–58

relationship between material interaction, material experience, art product, and mental health *59–61*
resilience 11, 12

salutogenesis 11
self-compassion 23
self-management 11, 13–14, 78, 86; in indication 70, 71; in step 4: Formulating 87
self-organization 11
sense of agency 21
sense of self 21
shared decision making 68
step 1: Observing 79–82
step 2: Analyzing 82–84
step 3: Interpreting 84–86
step 4: Formulating 86–87
structure of an art product 31, 51–52, *53*
structure of art-making *see* context of art-making
style of material interaction **41**, 42
subconscious *see* subcortical processes
subcortical processes 15–17, 21
sympathetic nervous system *see* autonomic nervous system

techniques and tools 6, *8*
Thematic Apperception Test (TAT) **35**, 37
therapeutic relationship 68–69
therapist 2, 68
transdiagnostic approach 10
transference 34

variation 53–56
vitality forms 21

World Health Organization (WHO) 11

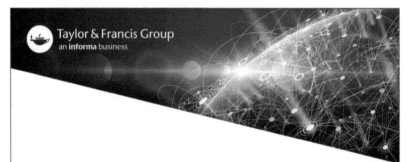

Taylor & Francis Group
an **informa** business

Taylor & Francis eBooks

www.taylorfrancis.com

A single destination for eBooks from Taylor & Francis
with increased functionality and an improved user
experience to meet the needs of our customers.

90,000+ eBooks of award-winning academic content in
Humanities, Social Science, Science, Technology, Engineering,
and Medical written by a global network of editors and authors.

TAYLOR & FRANCIS EBOOKS OFFERS:

A streamlined
experience for
our library
customers

A single point
of discovery
for all of our
eBook content

Improved
search and
discovery of
content at both
book and
chapter level

REQUEST A FREE TRIAL
support@taylorfrancis.com

 Routledge
Taylor & Francis Group

 CRC Press
Taylor & Francis Group